"GROWN UPS ARE REALLY STUPID"
What Children in Distress Teach Us

Doctor Daniel Rousseau

"Grown Ups are Really Stupid"

What Children in Distress Teach Us

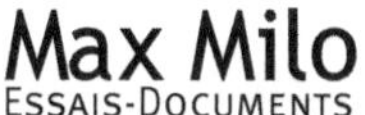

Max Milo
Essais-Documents

Max Milo Éditions
Collection Essais-Documents, Paris, 2023
www.maxmilo.com
ISBN : 978-2-31501-225-1

PREAMBLE

Early childhood remains unknown territory, even though we've all been there for a long time. We passed through it without looking at the landscapes or capturing the images, no doubt too preoccupied as we were with simply living and surviving. In the light luggage of our childhoods, we retain few tangible memories of this moving journey.

And yet, when we come across a little man, by some mysterious vibration of the soul, we immediately adapt to him, to the exact capacities of his age, to the obvious needs dictated by his dependence, finding under the fresh snow the trail we've walked a thousand times and our tracks still virgin. The foreign territory of his inner life becomes accessible to us again, as we respond without hesitation, as if we were once again permeable to this world of unspeakable emotions. In the moment, we perfectly perceive its relief, climate and colors. Yet words fail to describe the panorama.

Early childhood is a world of tender or violent, but fleeting emotions, whose perception, acute at this age, slowly fades. Indeed, when the time comes for feelings, words and memories, they are written in bold letters on the parchment of life, covering up the delicate primordial weave of emotions, like a palimpsest.

Deciphering the palimpsest?

.

Terra incognita

I'm a child psychiatrist. For the past twenty years, one day a week, I've left the quiet comfort of my consulting room to visit a children's home.

The very young children in distress who were taken in were a source of amazement and bewilderment to me, but I also learned a great deal from them. They had all been victims of acts unimaginable both in terms of their age and their seriousness: attempted infanticide, physical and psychological violence, neglect and abandonment, sexual abuse. The disastrous family living conditions they had faced prior to their admission further clouded the picture.

It took me twenty years of hindsight to realize that these situations, beyond the limits of the extreme, offered a formidable insight into the human being's relationship with his or her offspring, whether as a parent, a childcare professional, or simply as a citizen. But the dramatic stories of these little ones are as much about parenting as they are about a society's level of civilization. These abused children also question what is human in man.

The horror and abjection to which some of these children have fallen victim, even at the hands of their own parents, raises the question of the limits with which every father and mother is confronted. Where do we draw the line between tenderness, inappropriate confidences and sexual abuse? Where do we draw the line between authority, corporal punishment and violence? What's the difference between educational duty, exaggerated demands and psychological violence?

This brings us to another debate. If the actions of these children provoke horror or disgust in us, it's because we feel them to be the antithesis of ourselves. But how can we be sure? Between unworthy parents and the "good parents" we'd like to be, is there continuity or a break? And if there is a barrier, how does it rise up inside each of us? What guarantee do we have of its solidity? This raises questions about culture.

The ancients defined a barbarian by his cultural and geographical remoteness. A barbarian was someone who lived with strange customs, on the fringes of the Empire, far from civilization. They had to be protected and defended against. But contemporary history has dramatically demonstrated, beyond the realms of possibility, that barbarism inhabits man at the very core of ideologies as well as at the most intimate level of individuals. You don't have to go far from home to see its shadows lurking. Barbarity can also make its bed in the heart of the family.

The true nature of man is sometimes revealed most clearly in extreme situations. I observed how the dramatic nature of these children's situations, on both a vital and psychological level, acted as an amplifier, multiplying tenfold the strength of their emotions and the specificity of their expression. This magnifying glass effect brought to light psychic phenomena common to all children, but which go unnoticed in most of those whose development is happily banal. What was most astonishing was to observe that what manifested itself as a singular character, specific to each of them, carried with it a universal dimension peculiar to childhood, but which was only noticed with such acuity and obviousness in these extreme and very particular circumstances.

These foster children, growing up apart from their parents, but under the watchful eye of experienced professionals, can also reveal to us in a luminous way how the little human being constructs himself. What more astonishing and surprising field of research than to see these little beings structuring their relationship with others, expressing themselves with their bodies, developing their intelligence and feelings, shaping their identity, affiliating with their parents, asserting themselves as individuals or creating their own representation of the world: becoming human beings.

They also reveal unsuspected resources. Some manage to rise above their traumas, to grow up despite difficult parents, and to regain confidence in adults. Others even manage to develop compassion for their hopeless parents.

I invite you on a journey between wonder and horror.

The children featured on these pages have all been taken in by a nursery run by Aide Sociale à l'Enfance. These are permanent care facilities for babies and young children entrusted to the general council of a département, by court order in most cases, and by the parents themselves in a very small proportion.

These nurseries, formerly known as "hospitals for foundlings", were founded by Louis XIV to meet the State's obligation to take in abandoned children, a task that overwhelmed charitable organizations were no longer able to fulfill. This decision by the State, the starting point of a twofold historical movement - the organization of institutionalized infant care, followed by medical research to provide them with the best possible care - was initiated in France and then developed in identical fashion in all the major European nations, and later in the New World. It was in these nurseries that pediatrics and child psychiatry were forged until the middle of the 20th century.

In France, three hundred thousand children under the age of twenty benefit from child protection measures, half of which are placements. Children under the age of six account for a third of admissions to child welfare services.

A hidden world, disturbing, suspicious and unknown, but rich in unsuspected humanity.

The fifteen or so stories that make up this book are certainly not exhaustive of the variety of situations encountered, but they do enable us to grasp the spirit that drives this nursery: to observe these children, with finesse and respect, in order to respond in the most appropriate way to their real emotional and psychological needs.

Underlying these stories is the truly exceptional work of nursery assistants, childcare assistants, nursery nurses and educators, whose skills and dedication are remarkable.

1.

DAVID IS LOOKING FOR HIS FATHER

Misleading a child about his parentage can drive him mad

From the fax machine at the nursery comes a civil status certificate changing the surname of four-year-old David. His mother had contracted a sham marriage with a foreigner, no doubt for mercenary reasons, while maintaining an affair with the man who was to become David's father. But when he was born, the child bore the name of this unknown stranger, and his real parents soon separated. After her divorce, his mother began proceedings to disavow paternity, and David found himself torn between three surnames: that of his fictitious father, his mother's maiden name and his father's name. The change in civil status was expected and well known. A simple administrative document to be archived in the file.

The nursery nurse in charge of the service files it away, but decides to suggest to the mother and child that they meet with me and the young psychologist on the service to discuss the name change. She quickly informs me of this appointment, without having the time to tell me more about what prompted her to make this decision, perhaps because it was based on a gut feeling, with the instinct that comes from experience, without being able to justify it explicitly.

On the appointed day, the four of us meet up for a fairly conventional appointment to inform the little boy of his new name, which he already knew. It's almost noon, the mom arrives a little late - she's held up at work, she apologizes - and everyone gets ready for a fairly quick appointment. A simple formality.

David sits quietly on his mother's lap, and she trivializes the event: David had asked to be given the same name as his little brother, i.e. their mother's maiden name. I take the opportunity to ask about David's father, whether she has kept in touch, whether her son knew him: the usual questions. Yes, of course, even though they didn't live together, David's father Jeremy took a lot of care of him during his first year, and she entrusted him to him regularly. She was married at the time and he was unable to recognize the child. But David knows the first and last name of his real father, Jérémy Cousseau[1]. He lived at her parents' home in a small village, and she often visited them before meeting her new partner. Obviously, they remained on good terms, but didn't keep in touch. Just life!

David, who until then had been listening quietly, starts to get agitated, gets off his mother's lap and runs into the room. He asks:

---

1. A dummy name, but one whose consonance can be articulated with this story.

- What's his name? Jérémy? Jérémy Groussin (an educator by that name[2]), Jérémy Rousseau?

- No, Jérémy Cousseau," replied his mother.

David listens to nothing, walks around the room, picks up a teddy bear and, while placing it rather violently on my lap, says:

"Here you go! It's a Jeremy!"

He's already gone again, gets excited, finds another, then another, and starts the same merry-go-round again, each time giving them the same name. Then, in an overflow of motor agitation, he grabs like a vine a garland of Santas hanging from the window curtains, a forgotten vestige of recent festive season. The garland gives way and, brandishing the Santas like a banner, he leaps in all directions. Like a whirlwind, David runs around the room and deposits the fruit of his raid on the pile of stuffed toys already in my lap.

This scene of verbal play on homonyms and the accumulation of figurines of fathers that he addresses to me is a beautiful staging of the imaginary outburst that invades him and mobilizes all his energy: what name to put on his father? What face to put on that name?

- I believe, madame, that David is questioning us and trying to find out more about his father.

And his mother gets tangled up in vague justifications:

- As I said, we didn't part angry, but I haven't heard from him, and then he had to change his cell phone. I'm sure he hasn't moved, but I'm afraid to go there because his parents didn't like me. And they have vicious dogs.

Finally, she reveals the truth:

---

2. Same comment.

1. David is Looking for his Father

- My lawyer told me I was safe because his father didn't recognize him, but I wouldn't want him to have any rights over the child.

But she doesn't go so far as to state the real reasons for her reluctance. She has been sentenced to prison for the severe abuse and neglect of her two children in dramatic circumstances from which she failed to protect them. David and his little brother's lives were saved only by the good fortune of having come across the insight and presence of mind of a gendarme and a nursery nurse. I sometimes explain to young doctors who come to the nursery for training that we only see children who are still alive, which may sound cynical, but it's the exact truth: for the dead, it's too late!

From his window, a former gendarme had seen a young man playing soccer with a two-year-old child. *Playing* was inaccurate. He was shooting the ball violently at the crying child. Fortunately, the pensioner alerted social services. The nursery nurse, dispatched to the child's home, noticed bruises on the child and managed to convince the parents to hospitalize him. But her gaze was also drawn to the very large head of the four-month-old baby sleeping in a cradle. Worried, she took him in too. The eldest child, David, had several skeletal fractures, some recent, others healed a few weeks ago, proving repeated injuries. They had obviously not been treated. His younger brother suffered from two voluminous brain haematomas, one older than the other, implying at least two successive traumas. This explained the visible deformation of his skull.

It was these events that had prompted the brothers' placement in the nursery two years prior to this appointment. David's real father could therefore have every chance of getting his son back if he so requested. And his mother had preferred to keep her son in the dark, hiding the identity of this father from him, rather than risk losing custody of him. She had chosen to give priority to her right of enjoyment - in the legal sense of the term - over the child, even if it meant preventing him from knowing his father, and thus sacrificing her son's needs and rights to her desire to possess him.

During this name-change appointment, as it turned out, David's agitation over the question of his father's physical knowledge and his vocal play on homonyms made it abundantly clear that he had been searching for his identity for what must have been a very long time. This encounter threw light on an enigma that kept coming up whenever I came across David in the nursery corridors.

Systematically, this intelligent child, who despite his young age already had a good grasp of language, would call me "Monsieur Dinosaure" from the age of three, or name a dinosaur figurine he was brandishing at me "Monsieur Rousseau", which could have passed for provocation. I'm not young, but I'm not prehistoric. David knew his father's surname, which had the same consonance as mine, but he himself bore the name of a complete stranger. His ease with language meant he could play on permutations and make puns. And this passion for identity, in the sense of suffering, compelled him to torture words and thus also the name that represented me, close to that of his father. Dinosaure is merely a sort of spoonerism or phonetic anagram of Daniel Rousseau, and has nothing to do with me personally, but says everything about David's imaginary frenzy, devoted to an incessant quest for his identity and the shape of words, especially family names. What's

1. David is Looking for his Father

my father's name, who does he look like? This child had not only been physically abused, he had also been subjected to the imaginary torture of the search for the meaning of names, due to his mother's refusal to give him the key, for fear of losing custody of her son.

A few months later, during a discussion with the child welfare worker in charge of the family - David was in foster care at the time - the nursery team shared their concerns about the child's psychological difficulties linked to his mother's intransigent stance. This concern gained ground: the mother eventually asked this professional to help her write a letter to David's father.

A few weeks ago, maintenance work on the nursery sandpit unearthed a prehistoric animal in what are admittedly fairly recent geological strata. One of the nursery teachers, who remembered the story, recognized it as David's dinosaur, the one he carried around everywhere, naming it after me. She took him in and gave him to me. I kept it on my desk for a few days, but my little patients all wanted it. Such a beautiful prehistoric piece is not a toy. It is now enthroned on the shelf of my library.

The International Convention on the Rights of the Child specifies that at birth, the child has the right to a name[3]. The name given is not a fanciful name, but one that places the

---

3. "The child shall be registered immediately after birth and shall have the right from birth to a name, the right to acquire a nationality and, as far as possible, the right to know and be cared for by his or her parents", *International Convention on the Rights of the Child*, 1989, article 7.1.

child in a line of descent, with precise rules specific to each national legislation[4].

Sometimes it's impossible to know a child's parentage at birth: when a child has been abandoned, for example, and then adopted. The child nevertheless has the right to know bits and pieces of his or her history, however tenuous they may be. The imaginary construction of the child's filiation - which in this case is twofold, natural and adoptive - will revolve around a few signifiers, a few images in a way, which he or she will agglomerate into a single story that only he or she can compose. His adoptive filiation is recorded in the civil register, so it's no secret. It's better for his parents to reveal it to him - the sooner, the better - than for it to be discovered by chance during an administrative procedure at the age of majority, for example, as I once saw. This is guaranteed to have a disastrous effect on the child's trust in his parents, and to wreak havoc on his psyche.

Revealing your true parentage to a child, tactfully of course, is a declaration of love. We have longed for you, you have come to fulfill that longing, and we are proud to have you as our child. It's a declaration that expects nothing in return. From his parents, it's confirmation that they've recognized him as their child. It's him and not someone

---

4. "When a child's filiation is established with regard to both parents at the latest on the day the child's birth is declared, or at any time thereafter, but at the same time, the parents choose the child's surname: either the father's surname, or the mother's surname, or their two surnames together in the order chosen by them, up to a maximum of one surname for each. In the absence of a joint declaration to the civil registrar mentioning the child's choice of name, the child takes the name of the parent whose filiation is established first, and the name of the father if filiation is established simultaneously with regard to both parents", *Civil Code*, article 311-21.

else, even if he wasn't born of them. And that this bond is irrevocable and unconditional. The child cannot grow up serenely without this priceless, free, all-risk insurance.

In children who are still very young, rationality and concern for the plausible have not yet altered the spontaneity of their emotional expression. They still have the ability to dream the world, and the poetic inventions of their arrival among men are extraordinary. It's this period, when their minds are still open to everything, that is the most propitious for these delicate announcements.

In other circumstances, for example in the case of gamete donation, the filiation displayed in the civil register reveals nothing of the intimate or medical history of the child's procreation. However, the time will come when his parents will tell him, out of respect for him, that he was the fruit of their love, but a fruitful one aided by a gift. The child needs to have this information, in the event of subsequent genetic counseling, for example. But this information can come quite late, when pride and the pleasure of living together have knitted solid bonds. It can be as early as the first requests for "technical" information on sex life and procreation, around the age of reason, but well before the onset of adolescence. And there's no need to go into detailed medical techniques. The child doesn't have to identify with a sperm straw or a glass test tube, but with the desire of his parents to welcome him.

When quality bonds are forged, when the parents' affection is a love that leaves the child free to think and express himself, the child's response is often astonishing and wonderful. But it comes later, in a moving impromptu moment, in an unpredictable form that leaves parents speechless.

2.

"Amélie! The Judge hasn't Heard a Thing!"

Listen up: a child's body can talk!

If you know this little girl, you can imagine the scene: a dialogue of the deaf in the children's judge's chambers. But the judge kindly asks Amélie :

"It's been reported to me that you're saying everywhere, to your teacher, in your foster home, to your psychologist, that you don't want to go to your parents' house for the weekend anymore. Can you give me your opinion on this?"

Silence. Amélie, a pretty blond eight-year-old, stares intently into the eyes of the juvenile judge, listening attentively. You'd expect her to respond, her pupils are so bright, but she remains silent and her face, contrasting with her sharp gaze, is filled with a timid, frozen smile. Were it not for her eyes, her expression might appear impassive and smooth. The judge, who has known Amélie's situation since she was a child, takes her time, puts her at ease and insists:

"It's not the first time I've heard you ask for this, but your parents are very insistent. Together with their lawyer, they're demanding that this right of access and accommodation be maintained. I can't suspend or reduce it without you giving me your opinion, here, between us, in the privacy of this office, with no other adults to influence you. I have a duty to make a judgment based on good reasons."

And Amélie, in the silence that settles in, lets out powerful borborygms and then sonorous farts. A real concert. But her mouth says nothing. And the judge, ushering into her chambers the professional in charge of her situation at the Child Welfare Office, adds:

"I'm sorry, but I haven't heard anything and I can't rule on a reduction of the right to accommodation. Amélie hasn't told me anything..."

Decency, no doubt, makes the judge pause, but she continues:

"... on the other hand, I was treated to a wind concert. I wouldn't have known Amélie as a shy, reserved little girl, I would have taken offense. Perhaps she was a bit disturbed today. We'll revisit all this at the next hearing."

Amélie had arrived at the nursery eight years earlier, aged just one month, after three weeks in paediatric intensive care. She had suffered severe abuse at the hands of her psychotic mother, immediately after a very short stay in the maternity ward. Amélie had nearly fifteen fractures all over her skeleton. It's a miracle that she survived the abuse. Her father, absent at the time of delivery, returned home a week or so later, but ended up taking Amélie to hospital when she cried incessantly and multiple haematomas were discovered. Her delusional mother was never able to explain much of what she had done: she felt her daughter wasn't eating enough, so she hit her. "The child must eat, the child must eat", she kept repeating.

Some schizophrenic mothers find it impossible to imagine the otherness of the other, which is even more pronounced if that other is a baby. Too helpless to perceive an infant's emotions, unable to feel their child's real needs, they have no other recourse than to invent a behavior, constructed not by adapting to the perceptible needs of this little being, but by reconstructing disparate memories of their own childhood experiences. They project this maternal fiction, completely divorced from reality, onto their baby, but without any coherence with its situation, real age or level of development. A young patient, after a visit to the nursery, will tell the nursing staff that she saw her baby, just a few weeks old, walking. Another will ask her infant of less than a year how his morning at school went. Or the mother who, during a visit to her youngest child only a few months old, starts reading him a long story from a thick storybook and gets angry when he looks away. Yet another mother who's angry that the big winter coat she bought two weeks ago at the summer sale hasn't been worn by her six-month-old little boy. It's August! Impossible to get her to listen to reason. She leaves with the clean coat, which she washes anyway. No dialectic possible!

This kind of misunderstanding can be dangerous, even fatal, for the child. This is undoubtedly what happened with Amélie's mother. Lean and lanky, probably a former anorexic, she was certainly traumatized as a teenager by this experience and by family pressure to feed herself. She reproduced a similar demand on this baby, increased tenfold by her delusional state, to the point of hitting her to

2. "Amélie! The Judge hasn't Heard a Thing!"

make her suckle more and better, to the point of breaking her into little pieces.

It took months of patience and dedication on the part of the nursery staff to reassure Amélie and bring her back to life. With her "physical" condition improving slightly, we turned our attention to her "psychological" condition, and the little girl was referred to a baby psychology unit in hospital. After several sessions of increasing crying, during which Amélie refused to leave the arms of her educator, the therapists gave up, explicitly accusing the nursery professionals of over-protecting this capricious child who, through their fault, could not accept separation.

That's when she came to me. She is eighteen months old. Amélie is sitting in the lap of her educator. Despite this secure position for any other child, she shows great tension. She hasn't abandoned herself to the knees that welcome her, but stands upright, her back very straight, just poised, on the lookout, as if pressed against an invisible surface. At the slightest noise, she jolts and may even stifle a sob. She keeps her fists closed. She doesn't smile, her tense, unmoving face giving her the air of a little old lady. Her gaze is piercing and severe, but she nevertheless tries to reassure herself by turning her head to regularly meet the gaze of this other woman who carries her.

Everything about her exudes suffering, anxiety and insecurity. She has been coming for consultation several times now, always accompanied by Sylvie, who looks after her at the nursery. The pattern of the session is always the same. She doesn't want to leave her caregiver's lap at any cost. To avoid rushing her, she sits on the carpet with her back to the wall, near the corner of the small room. The psychomotrician who receives her with me sits on the floor, within Amélie's reach. The grown-ups talk about her, talk to her and present her with toys, to no avail. Amélie remains camped on the knees that reassure her, refusing any contact or exchange other than a furtive glance and sometimes a little listening. She withdraws into herself and cries in silence.

Suddenly, a toy presented to her catches her eye. She reaches out to take it, touches it and then suddenly pulls back, crying, as if frightened by her gesture. The scene is repeated several times, giving us a key to the story.

Amélie is not simply experiencing the separation anxiety that is common at this age, when a child leaves its mother to go to someone less familiar. Amélie is persecuted by her own demand, terrified by her own need, annihilated by her own desire. Lacan[5] perfectly described the knotting together of these three dimensions of human satisfaction as a three-stage rocket. A need - thirst, for example - can be satisfied by a variety of beverages, from water to milk. Demand, on the other hand, is subject to an address: "I want you to give it to me." And desire is something in between, linking the satisfaction of a need to a demand for love. We see very clearly in young children, through their whims, how they play with these elements in search of proof of love: "I want to drink." Daddy gives a glass of water. "No, I want milk. Daddy gives milk. "No, I want Mommy to have it. Mommy gives the glass of milk." "No, I want a bottle." "Ah, but why are you still acting?" In truth, it's during these

---

5. MILLER (Gérard), "Besoin, désir, demande", in *Lacan*, Paris, Bordas, 1987, pp. 81-82.

little family comedies that children learn to play out the complex articulation of needs, desires and feelings.

For Amélie, this is not theater, but a tragedy with no way out. To be hungry and stricken for not suckling enough, to be thirsty and suffer martyrdom in her fractured body mobilized without regard, to scream and feel the torture of a brain that threatens to explode, compressed by the bruises. And all this for days on end. A vital need arises, and all hell breaks loose. Fifteen fractures don't heal in a few days, and leave residual pain when handling or moving for many months. Amélie has learned not to move and to be wary of her emotions, desires or needs as basic as feeding herself, which, if they no longer result in blows, can cause pain and awaken mortal anguish. Cry in silence, don't shout, move sparingly. What insecurity!

Next session: Amélie reaches for the toy, pulls back and cries. We talk about her anguish and terror of wanting something. Craving is life, it's movement, it's encounter. But for Amélie, craving awakens memories of pain, when need was a threat to her life. And we reassure the educators about their work: Amélie is not a capricious little girl, and they must continue to protect her. Amélie grabs the toy. Little by little, Amélie allows herself to live, to smile, to laugh, and much later to move and walk.

Amélie is now six years old. She's a little girl who still needs a lot of reassurance from adults she knows well and trusts to be able to express herself and be relaxed. Her integration into the school system has been difficult: she held the teacher's hand in the playground for several months, then stayed in her shadow for a while longer before managing to go out and play with the other children from time to time. As soon as a stranger appears in her environment, Amélie shuts up and puts her back against a wall.

She has adapted well to her foster family, where she has made immense progress. Her mother, of course, is still unable to perceive her daughter's otherness, and continues to project onto her her own delusional certainties about child-rearing. These are opinions so close to common discourse that it's difficult for an untrained observer to spot them as pathological. She would like to obtain accommodation for a weekend so that she can "be like all the other families and go to the seaside". She takes advantage of a consultation to try and sell her project. From a distance, pressed up against the wall, her hands hidden behind her back, Amélie listens and throws a "caca boudin" at her mother, accompanied by a loud fart. She's a shy, charming and polite little girl, and such an assertive reaction is highly incongruous with her. Amélie continues her litany, which she enriches - "Maman caca boudin" - with an insistence hitherto unimaginable for her. I point out to this mother that Amélie is always very insecure in encounters with her, and that she wouldn't be serene at home. She replies peremptorily that "all children love to go to the seaside and Amélie couldn't give up such a wonderful surprise". For a brief moment, I have the impression that Amélie, still pressed up against the wall, has managed to disappear into its thickness.

Amélie is seven years old. As a result of the abuse, the mother was stripped of her parental rights. However, through incomprehensible judicial circumstances, she was able to exercise her right to visit and live with the child, thus rendering the original judgment null and

2. "Amélie! The Judge hasn't Heard a Thing!"

void. As a result, Amélie now regularly finds herself at the home and in the care of this mother who was her torturer. Unintentional, of course, but how can you make a child understand? Amélie is terrified before every short weekend she spends with her parents. Every other weekend, she is seized with a high fever before leaving her foster family, leading to conflicts over the exercise of custody rights. The little girl observes and endures the strangeness of this woman who doesn't talk to her, doesn't ask her any questions about her life as a child, doesn't ask her opinion on anything, but takes care of her mechanically, without any apparent affect. She organizes her days with her daughter as if she were a puppet with no thoughts, feelings or will of her own. A child must eat this, do that, go to bed at such and such a time, must like to do this, must not like to do that. Amélie describes her visits to her mother as periods of suspended animation, when she is forced to remain passive and silent to avoid irritating her. Hence the social services' repeated request to the juvenile court judge to limit these visiting rights.

A few months later, at a new hearing, Amélie managed to express what was making her stomach ache, twisting her guts, tying her throat and preventing her from speaking, but that her stomach, her guts, her throat, had already been screaming: the terror of going to her parents' for the weekend. The judge finally heard her and reduced the visitation rights.

Children, for whom speech is still difficult, may have no other language than their bodies: sounds, cries, sighs, gestures, attitudes, tears, glances, escapes, refusals, oppositions, contortions, tensions, agitation or collapse, falls, absences or extreme vigilance, fever or tremors: an endless list. In Amélie's case, we can add immobility, stupor, silent weeping, muteness, erasure in the walls, winds, farts and borborygms.

Most grown-ups have forgotten the body language that was once theirs.

3.

Kevin Thinks He's a Bird

When grown-ups think they're goats

Her educator explained:
"I hold his hand tightly when he's at the top of the stairs; sometimes you'd be afraid he'd jump out and fly."

Kevin had just turned three when I first met him. He was an extremely odd child who hopped on the tips of his dewclaws and flew with his arms. He could also waddle around like a penguin, his wing stumps glued to his body. He approached others and explored objects by pecking at them with his hand folded at face level and two fingers pointed like a beak. His language was well-developed, though he could only conceive of conversing by cackling while accumulating avian concatenations, which was very curious: "Mommy-bird, Daddy-pigeon, Baby-chick." He only talked about birds, only cared about birds. Such an eccentric child is amusing for a moment and then, realizing that this is not playful behavior, leaves you feeling very uncomfortable.

Is it possible to be struck dumb at such a young age?

The educator continued:

"Her mother was picked up drunk on the public highway. Someone asked if she had children. That's when he was found in her home, alone, abandoned, in a deplorable physiological state, locked in a cage-bed. He was sixteen months old. Immediately placed in the nursery, he didn't respond to us, didn't ask for anything and didn't look at us. His face was tense, he never smiled, never met our gaze and threw himself backwards if we approached him. He rocked back and forth in his bed and didn't respond to any adult requests. We thought he was deaf. He had never seen a doctor since he was born. He was very anemic."

His mother came to see him a few times, but never again responded to his various requests.

For many months, I received Kevin the bird and was overwhelmed with piles of bird drawings, then bird families. The skies of his landscapes were always filled with "V"s, as other children put clouds. When he was five, he explained:

"There are birds in Mama Fabienne's house, I'd like to go to her house to look at the birds, Mama Fabienne, she doesn't want me anymore..."

Kevin suffered enormously from his mother's abandonment. Later, when he talked to me about his early childhood, he would say "when I was a pigeon..." or "when I was a bird...".

At school, he learned to write his first name, which he proudly spelled out for me as "K. E. OISEAU I. N." It was Hitchcockian: even the alphabet was invaded by birds.

Drama: Kévin had to change foster families when the first childminder with whom he had stayed for several years stopped working. The break-up rekindled his feelings of abandonment and plunged him back into a fundamental insecurity that invaded all his attachment points. If someone he had held on to let go of him, Kévin imagined that others would too. Once again, he became like a bird on a branch. So he asked me:

"If I leave Mama Cathy's - her childminder - will I still be able to come to your house?"

His interest in animals then became somewhat bizarre and morbid: "When a mygale is on you, you mustn't move, if it falls it might die."

Abandonment meant fall and death for him.

His school career remained chaotic, passing through various medical-vocational institutes. As a young adult, he was described as introverted, rude, very solitary and possibly violent, but managed to build a lasting emotional relationship with a young girl. Doubtless subject to auditory hallucinations that he tried to silence, he was hospitalized after piercing an eardrum with a carpentry tool in his apprentice workshop. He summed up his painful destiny at the time: "I don't want to have children. If I'm going to do what my mother did and abandon them, I can't do it. What's more, I wouldn't know how to look after them, so I don't want any."

It's not unusual to meet toddlers in the nursery who present themselves as wild children and sometimes, like Kevin, in an animal identification. These are children who have always been the victims of great emotional abandonment and neglect - closet children, children for whom the parents had only a minimum of physical attention, but no affective concern, most often in very deficient families, marked by mental illness and intellectual deficiency - even though they had been left in the care of their parents.

Observers are always amazed by the highly unusual behavior of these babies, whose cries - whether in tone, modulation, rhythm or reactivity to human presence - attitudes, postures, contacts and interests seem so very unhuman. These behaviors evoke a quirkiness of being that sometimes, according to the child, goes so far as to recall an animal. This zoological illusion allows us to cling to a familiar branch to dispel the feeling of vertigo provoked by the strangeness of the non-human. Nothing a child acquires is innate; it is only built through interaction with other humans. And when forced by the emptiness of his surroundings to survive almost alone, he produces an unheard-of, distorted way of being in the world.

One of these children had bitten another on the cheek so savagely, detaching a large flap of flesh, that pediatric surgeons had great difficulty admitting that it was a human bite, let alone that it was the bite of a young child.

Another, two-and-a-half-year-old Régis, has virtually no language, having lived with intellectually limited parents who fought violently in front of their son, but paid no attention to him. He gets around on all fours and barks like his only playmate. He's also a biter.

Seven-year-old Antoine, a restless child with a strange and disturbing sense of smell about people and things, tells me about his passion for dogs, his only topic of conversation apart from his adoration for his foster mother. He explains that, before being placed with this family, he lived with his parents in the doghouse to avoid being beaten by his father.

I also remember Oriane, kept lying in her crib by her mentally deficient and psychotic mother until she was placed in a home at the age of eighteen months. She showed considerable intellectual and motor retardation. At the age of two, she was just beginning to get around on all fours. This didn't stop her from being extremely aggressive. Her educators even compared her to an eagle. Without language, she had a piercing black stare, which was accentuated by a wrinkling of the nose when she thought she was being attacked. She would then swoop down on an adult or another child, grabbing them with her talons and biting them until they bled, even if it meant ripping off the skin.

Coming back to Kevin, he wasn't, of course, fed by birds, but the sight of captive birds in the room where he lived, abandoned in his cage-bed, was certainly a living, sounding landmark in his life as a recluse.

An abandoned child cannot survive on its own and dies quickly. Stories of children taken in by animals are nothing more than myths and legends, which have been around ever since man became sedentary and sought to "d'homme-stiquer" animals, as Lacan spelled it.

The fate of these children is always fabulous, which may have been one of the reasons for the custom of exhibiting[6] children in Greece and Rome. If a child survived the ordeal of abandonment, it was a sign that he or she was protected by the gods. It was therefore only natural that animals should come to his aid. In sixth form, we all learned the

---

6. "Exposing" a child was a term used until the middle of the 19th century to designate the act of depositing a newborn child in a public place in the hope of being taken in. In France, over six million children were abandoned in this way between the end of the 17th century and the middle of the 19th century.

story of the birth of Rome and the collection of Remus and Romulus by a she-wolf[7].

"After the birth of the two children, when the tyrant demanded their death, to whom did Fortune allow them to be delivered? It was not to a barbaric or savage servant, but to a compassionate and humane man, who had no thought of killing them. On the contrary, as there was a vast meadow on the banks of the river, bathed by its waters and shaded all around by trees that almost touched the ground, he deposited the children near a wild fig tree, which has since been called Ruminalis. Then there was a she-wolf who had just given birth, and whose udders were swollen and fat with milk. She herself was in need of relief, as her cubs had died. So she attached herself to the two cubs, presented them with her teats; and it seemed as if she became a mother a second time by getting rid of her milk."

Although this touching anthropomorphic description of the animal dates back twenty centuries, it's part of a very long tradition that goes back to ancient Egypt and probably to prehistoric times, as evidenced by the painted animals in ornate caves.

So it's hardly surprising that in the Greek Pantheon, the great Zeus himself was suckled by the Amalthea goat[8] and that Apollodorus[9] reports that Paris was suckled by a bear, as was Atalanta. King Cyrus was fed by a bitch; Telèphe, son

---

7. PLUTARCH, *Œuvres morales*, "De la fortune des Romains", chapter VIII.

8. "Let my song go forth from Jupiter! During the first night, I can see the star that hastened to Jupiter's cradle: this is the rising of the rainy sign of the Olenian Goat. She has her place in heaven for the price of the milk she has given." OVID, *Fastes*, V-111.

9. APOLLODORUS, Library: III, 12 5-6.

of Hercules, by a doe, and Semiramis by doves. Justin[10] tells us that Habis, grandson of Gargoris, was abandoned by his grandfather, but fed by various wild beasts and finally by a doe who "came to offer him her teats".

On the ceiling of the Opéra Garnier, Chagall's[11] depicts Daphnis and Chloe being fed by a goat and a sheep respectively. The epitome of anthropomorphism, Longus - the author of this ancient novel - tells us that the shepherd who took in Daphnis gave the goat that had saved the child a burial close to that of men: "I found him [Daphnis] abandoned by father and mother, suckled by one of my goats, whom I buried in the garden, after she had died her natural death, having loved her for what she had done as a mother to this child."

At the very beginning of the 19th century, the capture of the Sauvage de l'Aveyron, a child wandering in the woods, and his care by Dr. Jean-Marc Gaspar Itard at the Institut des sourds-muets du faubourg Saint-Jacques in Paris, aroused great public and scientific curiosity about wild children. Abbé Pierre-Joseph Bonnaterre, a professor of natural history in Rodez, wrote a historical note listing a dozen children said to have been found in the 16th and 17th centuries among animals including wolves, bears, sheep and oxen.

In nineteenth-century France, because of difficulties in recruiting a sufficient number of nannies to breastfeed the large numbers of abandoned infants taken in by children's hospitals, goats were used for this purpose in several

----

10. Justin's Universal History from Trogue Pompey.
11. Roman de Longus, 1st or 2nd century AD.

3. Kevin Thinks He's a Bird

towns. Dr. Montfalcon describes his experiences at the Hospices de Lyon:

"The size and shape of this animal's teats, the abundance and good qualities of its milk, the ease with which it can be trained to present its udder to the child, and the attachment it is likely to develop for the newborn, make it highly suitable for this purpose. We choose a young goat, which has only recently given birth, which is not in its first litter, and whose habits are gentle and peaceful. The milk of goats with white coats is virtually odorless. The child is placed on the ground, in a low cradle; and at the beginning of this mode of suckling, the servants take the greatest care to preserve the newborn from the animal's petulance and impatience. Although this type of nursing may have a few advantages, in a large hospital it can only be an exceptional solution."[12]

For his part, Abbé Gaillard adds:

"I'm talking about direct suckling by a goat. You can't fail to be touched by the way these good animals call their adopted children with their bleats, welcome them with their caresses, and lend themselves with astonishing docility to the needs, even the whims, of their infants. But this method requires a great deal of care, and can only be applied in exceptional cases. How do you keep a herd of two hundred goats in the middle of a big city, and the people you need to look after them? Let's face it, newborns get used to this type of feeding very well."[13]

---

12. TERME et MONTFALCON, *Histoire des enfants trouvés*, Paris, Paulin, 1840.

13. Abbé GAILLARD, *Recherches administratives, statistiques et morales sur les enfants naturels et les enfants trouvés*, Paris, Leclerc, 1837.

In the twentieth century, mankind moved away from nature and became *homo urbanus*, leading to an imaginary explosion of animal figures in children's literature and cinema. Animals have lost their wild or utilitarian character and have regained the roles of totemic figures they had at the dawn of humanity. Fictional characters such as Tarzan[14], Mowgli[15], or the lesser-known Saturnin Farandoul[16] - the story of a four-month-old baby adopted by orangutans, imagined in 1879 by Albert Robida - may well have been inspired by these mythological and historical tales.

This very long history of imaginary companionship between children and animals shows us that man has always questioned the boundaries between human and animal. Man has sought to define *his nature* between humanity and bestiality, between the intelligence of the *sapiens* and the cognition of the animal, in similarity or in opposition, and this, in all aspects of human life. The way we parent, father or mother, the way we raise our children, have not escaped this illusory process of zoomorphism.

I'm still amazed at the general credulity - and by all means, test your friends and family discreetly on the subject - of the belief that a young child could survive on the company of animals alone. Even today, this kind of story continues to fascinate, tapping into the public's candor.

---

14. From BURROUGHS (Edgar Rice), *Tarzan chez les singes*, translated from English by A. Lucyon, Paris, Fayard, 1912.

15. From KIPLING (Joseph Rudyard), *The Jungle Book*, Paris, Mercure de France, 1899.

16. *Jules Verne's Voyages très extraordinaires de Saturnin Farandoul dans les cinq ou six parties du monde et dans tous les pays connus et même inconnus* are available for free consultation on the BNF website: http://gallica.bnf.fr

3. Kevin Thinks He's a Bird

Misha Defonseca[17] finally admitted in 2008 that her autobiographical bestseller *Surviving with Wolves* - translated into eighteen languages and brought to the screen to great commercial success - which recounted her adoption by a pack of wolves in 1941, was pure fiction.

We might smile at such widespread popular naivety, but we should be wary of it. This ancient belief in the saving, nurturing and tutelary virtues of animals is still at work in today's families. Modern parents are careful never to leave their young offspring without the tactile and olfactory support of a bear, a lion or even a stuffed dolphin.

But a careful reading of the ancients leaves no doubt as to their opinion on the matter: its improbability. In these texts, ancient animal nannies were never more than the helpers of a benevolent shepherd, nymph or hunter. And none of the wild children listed by Abbé Bonnaterre were endowed with language. As for the goats in the children's hospitals, they were trained for this function. In conclusion, Thierry Gineste's book on *Victor de l'Aveyron, dernier enfant sauvage, premier enfant fou*[18] demonstrates the epistemological break introduced by Itard's work.

There is no humanity possible for a child outside the affection of his fellow human beings.

Kévin, who had never known human compassion with his parents, built a pseudo-humanity with animals. He became a bird.

---

17. "One of the monuments to the universal credulity of recent decades", according to surgeon Serge Aroles, who denounced this deception. "Misha Defonseca: tricher avec les loups", *L'Express*, February 29 2008.

18. GINESTE (Thierry), *Victor de l'Aveyron. Dernier enfant sauvage, premier enfant fou*, 1st ed. 1981, Paris, Hachette, coll. "Pluriel", 2011.

4.

CATHY SAVED BY MARIE-LO

Abuse has always existed, and so have foster families

Long before men thought of imitating them, the gods of Antiquity had their own child protection service. The poet Homer, the philosopher Plutarch, the historian Pausanias and the mythographer Apollodorus recounted their adventures, now forgotten and little-known. The most notable are certainly the actions of the Egyptian goddess Isis and the Greek goddess Thetis on behalf of divine children in danger.

Isis possessed three virtues: she could reinfuse life, she was a nurturing goddess and she had the gift of true speech.

Aphrodite, wife of the terrifying Typhon, gave birth in secret to a boy, whom she promptly abandoned for fear of her husband. Isis went in search of him, found him and took charge of feeding him; the child became her guardian and follower under the name of Anubis. It was with his help that she succeeded in embalming Osiris. Indeed, when the terrible Typhon had, out of jealousy, cut up Osiris, Isis' brother and husband, into fourteen pieces, Isis searched for the various parts of his body, which she recovered scattered all over the world, except for the phallus, which she was unable to find and made into a clay imitation. Having collected these pieces, she embalmed them, wrapped them in bandages, creating the first mummy, and breathed life into it. Isis also gave birth to a son "born prematurely and weak in the lower limbs", whom she cared for and who became the little god Harpocrates. Finally, Isis, says the fable, wears an amulet around her neck, the name of which is "true speech", for, adds the philosopher, no attribute among those that man has received from nature is more divine than speech.

Plutarch also explains that his compatriots associate Isis and Thetis as mythological nannies who take in and nurture sickly babies. Thus, Thetis and Eurynome, sea goddesses, took in Hephaestus, a crippled baby thrown down from Olympus by his parents Zeus and Hera. Hephaestus remained a hunchbacked, lame god, much to the hilarity of the other inhabitants of Olympus. He conceived an eternal affection and gratitude for his comforters, the measure of divine time.

To be the nurturer, to bring together the scattered pieces of body and spirit, to give life and give the gift of a true word - these are the extraordinary tasks carried out with humble and precious devotion by some foster families who receive the care of young, battered babies.

One-year-old Cathy is entrusted to Marie-Lo. Cathy had arrived at the nursery a few weeks earlier, and we quickly realized that she was in a very serious state of dereliction, and that it was absolutely essential to provide her with intensive emotional resuscitation care, for which living in the community was not a satisfactory solution.

Given Cathy's alarming condition, it was both a necessity and a gamble to entrust her to a childminder. We were well aware of the heavy workload this would entail for her, and the exhaustion that would ensue if Cathy's progress proved too stagnant. Caring for babies in such mental distress requires a great deal of determination to fight against the despairing and destructive spiral represented by the absence of gratifying emotional feedback from the child or too little progress. This can quickly discourage and demobilize even the most hardened. The risk of a foster placement failure could not be ruled out, but we really had no choice.

Little Cathy is indifferent to everything, and the world seems non-existent and uninhabited to her. Cathy doesn't look for people to look at her, nor does she respond to those who do. Nor does she react to noises, nor does she respond to sound solicitations, which she seems to ignore. From her stroller in the street, she looks at nothing, neither the joyful wriggling of the neighbor's dog, nor the roar of the monster swallowing garbage in its gaping maw. When a loud noise occurs, she doesn't even flinch. In the house, she gets around on all fours and may bump into bodies as if they were only there to fill the space. She allows herself to be passively force-fed, putting her fingers in her mouth to pull out bits of food that she then manipulates as strangeness. She doesn't call out for her needs or desires to be met, but can scream in a nagging way for no apparent reason and with nothing to soothe her. An absent, inaccessible baby, beyond the reach of the living.

Her mother took care of her physically, but shunned emotional exchanges with her daughter. She was a woman pervaded by rituals centered on housework, hygiene and cleanliness. Her home was spotless, and so was her baby. Cathy was cleaned, washed, washed, changed, dressed, bottle-fed, put to bed, lifted, lifted, turned over, wiped, wiped, cleaned, polished, moved in a stroller. Her mother organized these tasks according to immutable rituals determined by fixed schedules that took no account of the child's reality, needs or reactions. This mentally disturbed mother had been admitted with Cathy to a mother-child psychiatric hospital for a few months, in an attempt to help them establish a relationship. There, she invariably bathed Cathy at four o'clock in the morning, because "it was time", much to the annoyance of the staff, who were shocked that she would wake their daughter in this way. What's more, this washing ritual was devoid of any tenderness, as her mother couldn't bear to hold Cathy against her. To wash her, she held her at arm's length and kept her at a distance like a dirty, nauseating object. As for feeding her, whether her daughter was crying from hunger or still asleep, the bottle had to be taken at a fixed time, regardless of the child's perceptible needs. At three months, Cathy was smiling; at six months, her only expression was painful, mute grimaces or contortions of the arms and body. By a year old, she was an absent baby whose shrill cries to no one could be soothed. No amount of advice or remarks could change this mother's rituals.

This regime prevents the baby from establishing connections between the functioning of his body, his needs, and the beneficial occurrence of an adapted response, i.e. between the strangeness of the sensations of his internal machinery and the reassuring maternal word that baptizes them, granting them existence and geography. The result is a rapid disarticulation of the soul and dismemberment of the body, as surely as an executioner in the Place de Grève would execute his dirty work, quartering and then slicing with axe and horse.

So Cathy can hurt herself badly and still not show it. Sometimes she hits herself hard - you feel a shiver down your spine - but carries on as if nothing had happened, without flinching or crying. We've even seen her, in moments of great distress, actively slam her temple against the leg of a heavy table without letting on. This pain seems to be foreign to her, and its manifestations absent. The bone in her head certainly hurts, but she's not in pain, no longer in pain. This bodily sensation no longer belongs to her, because no one has collected it to give it value and consistency. Her mother, who undoubtedly never experienced this benevolent thoughtfulness for herself, didn't know how to pay attention to it, and no doubt didn't offer herself to these nursemaid's games of blowing on sores, singing a soothing little refrain or saying a few consoling words in the same way that kings touched the scrofula of the unfortunate or saints laid hands on the sick.

In 1801, Dr Itard described the same insensitivity to pain and the same phenomenon of disconnection of the senses and emotion in young Victor de l'Aveyron, discovered in the woods: "The child's eye was wandering and haggard. No doubt he could see, but he could not look. The loudest noises hardly seemed to strike his ear; a doorbell, a pistol shot, didn't make him turn around."[19]

---

19. GINESTE (Thierry), *Victor de l'Aveyron*, Paris, Hachette Littératures, 2004, p. 423.

At the nursery's service meeting, we talk about the strangeness of Cathy's behavior, about her broken body, her scattered emotions, her indifference to the human feelings of those around her, about Itard, Isis and Thetis.

Marie-Lo continues to observe this apparent anaesthesia of Cathy's body and worries: this little girl has no regard for herself. So she invents a whole stratagem to make the pain she observes in Cathy's body exist in her mind, but to which Cathy doesn't seem to be sensitive. If Cathy bumps into something, Marie-Lo shrieks "ouch! ouch!" and starts blowing and rubbing the bruised spot. Cathy, impassive and then astonished, watches this merry-go-round, which repeats itself with each new bump.

Cathy allows herself to be force-fed passively and mechanically. She shows neither hunger nor satiety, whatever the quantities ingested, and neither pleasure nor displeasure at the variety of the menu. Marie-Lo once noticed a slight retching. She interprets this as the end of the meal. She tells Cathy. Soon, Cathy, who remains very calm when she's hungry, starts to squirm when she doesn't want any more. Marie-Lo notices this and comments on her calm appetite, her little agitation and her desire to stop eating. Cathy has seized on this code, so there's no need to wait for nausea. Marie-Lo doesn't ask questions, but speaks enunciations: an immediate reading aloud of Cathy's bodily manifestations, consciously taking the risk of misinterpreting.

Marie-Lo explains: "I realized with Cathy that I had to be very receptive to the little signals she showed, which can be very different from those you'd expect from any other child. Once I've identified what seems to me to be one of these signals, always discreet, I name it and emphasize its significance, considering it to be of communication value.

Cathy probably doesn't mean anything by it, but I make this bodily reaction exist as a means of expression and show her that it has meaning for me."

Cathy's body becomes a dramatic space, with Marie-Lo directing, translating and commenting.

"It became a kind of reflex, I felt in Cathy's place, I thought in Cathy's place, I sounded in Cathy's place, I spoke in Cathy's place. A toy would slip out of her hand, and I'd cry out 'boom!' She seemed to like mashed potatoes, and I'd go 'hum! hum! c'est bon'. She'd open her mouth, and I'd say 'mam! mam! I want some'. I commented on the world, hers and ours. I commented aloud on her environment, the mashed potatoes in her mouth, the freshness of the water, the noise of the fridge, the absence of my daughters, the cooling wind, the return of my husband, the dazzling sun, the wobbling manhole cover, the flying leaf, and all the little events of daily life, so subtle that we no longer noticed them, but which she certainly perceived. And I named everything she did. Cathy, you're the one who took the ball out of my hand. Cathy, I can see you're hungry. Cathy, what progress: you're eating the cake all by yourself...

And I would invent little scenarios that I would repeat tirelessly. Every day, when I got back from a walk, I'd ring the letterbox and pretend to hit my head, adding a big 'bang' and rubbing my skull. No reaction from him. Three months, it took three months! But once, perhaps out of weariness or in too much of a hurry, I forgot to do it, and it was Cathy who said 'bang' to me as we walked past, rectifying my oversight. I might as well say it woke me up!"

Marie-Lo often takes Cathy for a walk in her stroller, where she finds peace of mind. Sitting in the direction of travel, Cathy watches the landscape unfold before her. Now, she's delighted to meet the neighbor's dog, whose mood is as cheerful and even-tempered as his master's: "Hello Cathy! Let's go for a walk!" Now Cathy follows with her eyes the hiccups and flutters of the antique tractor mowing the lawn, and worries when the noisy garbage truck arrives.

One day, Cathy turned to look at Marie-Lo and never left her side. It's hard to drive a stroller in these conditions, but Marie-Lo remembers the first few months, when Cathy ignored even her gaze. Soon, Cathy contorts her body and maintains this uncomfortable position, timidly reaching out for Marie-Lo's hand as she drives. Marie-Lo gives her a finger, Cathy takes it and keeps it. Even more difficult to steer the stroller in this position, but the moment is too precious. Marie-Lo relates this episode with emotion.

From now on, in the impromptu events of everyday life, Cathy will seek out this finger wherever it may be, and drown in Marie-Lo's eyes as she feeds her baby in the morning.

The arms like a cradle, the caressing voice, the scent of skin, the milk that sustains, the hand like a cuddle, a finger to hold, the warmth of the lap, the gaze that drinks in, quiet abandonment and peaceful emotions: the gentle presence, like an envelope. Cathy reconnected with the carnal perception of this tender incarnation, a veritable psychic placenta that conveys permanence and security, and gave her back the sensation of existing. Soon, little play rituals were added to these vital exchanges, prolonging and extending the time of the encounter. At the morning feed, Marie-Lo noticed that the ceremonial had to be immutable: the same place on the sofa, the bottle in the same position. Then Cathy introduced her own variations. Stop feeding, take the bottle and try to put the teat in Marie-Lo's mouth.

And then play with the face-shaped cupcake. Marie-Lo has to show the cake man's mouth, nose and eyes. Cathy takes it, lets Marie-Lo taste it and then finally eats it. First games and exchanges where Cathy experiments and separates what belongs to her and what belongs to Marie-Lo in a still visible confusion of emotions and images of self and other. Cathy has not yet achieved the perception of her undivided and different self from Marie-Lo, which will constitute the second deliverance: that of the psychic placenta. Cathy has invented another ceremonial. Now, when she stumbles, even slightly, she goes round all the family members so that everyone can blow on her boo-boo!

There's still a long way to go, but Cathy, the boneless celluloid doll, is back among the living. She has rediscovered a taste for the exchanges, gifts, words and tenderness that are the hallmark of human beings. But this care remains difficult, as these moments of grace can still be rare and isolated. Marie-Lo always expresses the feeling of having to deal with a foreign child with whom the continuity of the relationship is never assured. Cathy can relapse into her slump for no reason, and then everything has to be redone.

Cathy is now two and a half years old. Unless you know about it and have a professional eye, no one notices the little residual quirks in her behavior anymore.

Cathy has to meet her mother at the social center, the judge has decided. Marie-Lo accompanies her. It's the same every time: tension before the visit, then a silent separation as Cathy sinks into indifference until she is picked up again. This time too, Marie-Lo feels Cathy's body stiffen against her as they approach the visiting room where her mother is waiting. But just before they arrived,

Marie-Lo was surprised to hear Cathy say "scared!" very clearly, while clutching tightly at the collar of her garment with both hands. Cathy herself named this tense body, the anxiety she felt at having to leave Marie-Lo and find her sick mother.

The body that speaks, the emotion that deafens, the word that binds them together: Cathy has finally joined the territory of men, these speaking beings who count their inner and outer worlds. That which has no name does not exist. Without man, there would be nothing.

When you talk to Marie-Lo today about Cathy's long road back to our humanity and the incredible perseverance she has shown, and ask her what it was that kept her going all this time, waiting for Cathy's first real look, her first words, her first tender gestures, she simply replies that at the end of their first meeting in the nursery, Cathy, who had been completely indifferent until then, had caught her gaze for a split second:

"I attached myself to that fleeting sparkle in his eyes, telling myself that maybe I'd manage to reap more."

Once the spark had been lit, Marie-Lo blew on this almost cold ember and managed to revive Cathy: she succeeded in bringing the soul back into this little body.

To be the nurturer, to bring together the scattered pieces of body and mind, to reinspire life and give the gift of a true word: the heroic and unsung work of some foster families and the vocation of every parent.

The job of family assistant - foster family - is undoubtedly one of the most difficult jobs there is. It is not recognized for its true worth, and family assistants - despite the recent professionalization law[20] concerning them - are all too often regarded as mere collaborators in the child welfare system, even though they are its linchpins. Indeed, they are the ones who have access to the child, who confides in them, showing them the pain of existing and the joy of living. Without their presence and attention, it would be difficult to accurately assess the child's difficulties, as well as his or her progress. Foster families are the child's true spokespeople.

In a few rare departments, and in some specialized foster care services, they are now recognized as true professionals, participating as such in various meetings concerning the child and his or her family with other child specialists.

We still have a long way to go before they are given their rightful place.

---

20. Law no. 2005-706 of June 27, 2005 on maternal assistants and family assistants.

5.
"Yannick Builds Prisons for Himself"

You can try to forget your child, but he won't forget you.

Yannick questions his childminder.

\- Why didn't Mum come?

\- Mom got into a lot of trouble and the judge put her in jail.

Three-year-old Yannick can't quite imagine what it's like to be in prison, but he does notice the passage of time and the insistent absence of his mother, who no longer comes to visit him. Weeks go by, and Yannick asks more questions.

\- Where's Mom?

\- In prison, she can't get out to see you.

\- Does she eat at the prison?

\- Of course we feed him.

\- Is she sleeping at the prison?

\- Don't worry, Mommy has a bed over there.

Yannick certainly remembers the wandering life he experienced with his mother before her placement, with no security from one day to the next, neither for food nor lodging.

- What's prison like?

- It's like a really big house with bars. You can't get out.

The time without seeing Maman lengthens again. Yannick's behavior changes. Hitherto an easy-going, gentle and gratifying little child, he begins to clash, lose his temper and storm around his foster family. He becomes impatient and demands, in an angry voice and imperative tone:

- When's Mum getting out of prison!

Yannick has become unrecognizable. A true rebel, with a hard, provocative look, he now invents great nonsense. Nothing satisfies him, and he rejects everything that used to please him. He ends up destroying his belongings and breaking his own toys, even the ones he holds dearest.

The situation gets even worse. The naturally sweet and quiet little boy is now attacking the woman who looks after him and to whom he is tenderly attached: his nursery assistant. No doubt finding it distasteful that "Lolo", as he calls her, passionately tends the flowers in his garden beds, Yannick carefully cuts off all the buds in this spring, which is shaping up to be without Maman. Unhappy that Lolo is also taking care of the little girl he has taken in, she gets a few nasty kicks.

His exasperation escalates even further: in his tantrums, he now goes so far as to hit Lolo. His mother fails him, but it's to his nanny that he addresses his frustration at being left behind. On the outside, at school, all is well; the other grown-ups are not concerned by this private affair.

Punishments obviously only make things worse, fueling his disenchantment and disenchantment, and "Lolo" doesn't know what to do anymore, becomes exhausted and anxious. The child welfare worker, trained "the old-fashioned way", thinks there's no point in seeing a psychologist or child psychiatrist. He's too small. Lolo doesn't mind hearing this; in fact, she thinks she's guilty. Lolo, who took great care of Yannick, the suffering baby she took in when she was very young, readily admits her difficulty in containing him - "before, I didn't need to scold him" - and blames herself for her helplessness. The foster placement, which had been working well, turned sour, and worse, vitriolic. Put in a difficult position by Yannick, with no support from the educator, and no solution proposed, Lolo feels she is in perdition, and keeping this child in her home is in danger.

At the staff meeting, this competent childminder looks desperate, at the end of her rope. She began to question her professional abilities and wondered whether she might just give up. It was then suggested that she meet me and Yannick.

As soon as the introductions are made, Yannick rushes to the box of figurines and brings to life a few old plastic fossils, dinosaurs that immediately start fighting and biting each other very savagely in an outburst of aggressiveness - with *Jurassic Park*, Steven Spielberg has consigned wolves to the ranks of antiques:

"He's mean, we'll put him in a cage. He's bad, we'll put him in jail - and turning to me - please, build me a jail!"

I build a prison-cage with two cubes and three pieces of wood.

Yannick lashes out at the dinosaurs, screams at them, throws them off with glee, organizes a punitive expedition to capture them, then locks them up in the prison:

"Naughty, naughty, not pretty!"

We agreed with Yannick that he would come back the following week to talk about dinosaurs.

But this time, dragons will be unleashed in a merciless war.

"Dragons should be caged because they're evil. No, they shouldn't! You have to put them in jail."

I'm building a prison. Yannick observes my work and comments in the learned voice of an expert who advises and orders:

"It's just a tiny little house, it's not a real prison, you have to make a big prison-house."

Yannick is certainly right: dragons are dangerous and difficult to lock up, they fly and they breathe fire! So I go ahead and build higher, thicker walls.

"Mom, she's mean, she doesn't come to see me, we have to put her in jail."

His mom wrote him a letter expressing her regrets at having done something stupid and consequently depriving Yannick of his presence. But he refused to listen when Lolo read the letter to him.

Accompanied by the child welfare worker, Yannick was able to visit his mother in prison. The educator reports that it was a disappointing visit for Yannick, as his mother remained rather distant from him and was not very demonstrative. It was a rather formal visit, without much affection or affection being exchanged, according to him.

At the next appointment, I ask Yannick about the visit. Silent for a while, he finally replies: "They're sad in the prison."

He looks worried. He'll play unconvincingly with dinosaurs and a doll lost in prehistoric times. He puts them all in prison, but soon asks me to build a hospital too.

I'm amazed at its relevance! Yannick recognized his mother's state of psychological incapacity, which he had been confronted with and involved in continuously for the first two years of his life, prior to his placement. As a result, he has acquired a finesse of psychological observation - how is Mum this morning, this afternoon, this evening? - which already far exceeds that of the professionals around him. They see only indifference and lack of attention, where Yannick reads psychological suffering and emotional apathy. At the tender age of three and a half, Yannick came across and recognized a distress even greater than his own, that of his mother, deeply depressed, so little expressive in her affections and very bruised by her inability to be, to be a mother among other things.

So we build a hospital. Yannick fetches the doll from the prison and takes it by ambulance to the hospital.

This renewed concern for his mother has been nagging at him. The visit to the prison rekindled the chaos.

Now Yannick is worried. He doesn't want to leave Lolo, doesn't want to leave her in the morning, asks her a hundred times if she'll be back to pick him up from school, worries about her lateness. He won't leave her side and won't let her out of his sight in the house. He cries and panics every time Lolo's husband or one of her children leaves the house.

Or Yannick may show great aggression towards Lolo through rebellious outbursts in which he laughs in her face and makes fun of everything. Lolo has even had to isolate him in the garage. He can also sink into the darkest anxieties. He talks about death, worries about the objects he puts in the garbage can or, on the contrary, throws them in with violence. Is he himself a disposable object? Then his worries about being separated from Lolo return, invading family life.

Yannick returned to see his mother in prison. This time, the visit went more smoothly, with a real reunion between Yannick and his mom. She was clearly feeling better. Yannick came back reassured and calmed, less worried about her. His behavior has calmed down and his periods of opposition have completely disappeared.

For the first time, Yannick agreed to come alone to a session with me. We even played hide-and-seek. Not for long, as Yannick was quick to call me to tell me where he was hiding, for fear that I wouldn't find him, hidden behind a green plant or under my office desk.

He wants a piece of paper to write on. He draws Lolo and her earrings. When he finds her, he says:

"I love you Lolo."

Lolo and her husband had to go away for a weekend and entrust Yannick to another family. They were careful to reassure him and let him know when they would be back.

"We're not abandoning you, we'll be back for you on Monday."

But on the way back, Lolo and her husband are treated to their own festival of kicks and tantrums. After the distress of feeling abandoned by his mother, Yannick is now worried that Lolo might abandon him too.

Yannick lets us see this strangeness and incongruity in the eyes of adults: a child who believes he's in danger of being abandoned may react with rage and attack the very adult he fears being separated from. In our grown-up logic, this seems completely counterproductive, as we believe that bonds of affection are built on wisdom or promises. If you're wise, you'll get an image! If you're not wise, we'll put you in a boarding school!

For the child, the fear of abandonment is measured in terms of self-preservation. To be abandoned is to be in mortal danger. Faced with such vital circumstances, adults' moral notions - wisdom, respect, constraint, or even blackmail and promises - seem derisory in this all-out fight for life[21].

Lolo senses Yannick's distress and fear of abandonment. She tries to reassure him:

"You're ours now."

At the next appointment, he finds a sheet of paper.

He draws a circle, two eyes, a nose and a mouth.

He's talking to himself, ignoring my presence.

He takes another sheet and draws Lolo with her earrings, then adds another character. Still ignoring me, he tells Lolo about his drawing, as if in a play:

He points to the second character in the drawing, Gigi, the nanny's husband.

He then draws Sarah, the oldest of the nanny's daughters, who is a young adult:

---

21. It is a common observation that the first feeling of grief is hatred for the deceased, because he or she has abandoned the person who loved him or her, and the latter is deprived of his or her love object. Children at risk of abandonment anticipate the loss, and express their hatred for the object of love before the event occurs. A double penalty then befalls these children: in addition to the anguish of the loss, they run the risk of rejection due to the behavioral problems that emerge. For them, it's a downward spiral. *At the very least,* this phenomenon can also be observed in small children who have been left in care longer than usual, and who "sulk" for a few minutes, sometimes a day or two, when their parents return. Separation anxiety is just a "degraded version" of this psychic mechanism.

5. "Yannick Builds Prisons for Himself"

"I love you" he addresses the portrait of the young woman and still snubs me.

He ignores me, but makes me a witness to this intimate mystery: what clearer declaration of love and what clearer request for love from the family that welcomed him!

His mother was released from prison. The following week, he tells me:

"I don't like Mommy, she didn't come to visit... She has a boo-boo, she broke her leg. I want to draw Mommy."

He drew her with a circle, two lines for the legs and two lines for the arms, one for the mouth and two dots for the eyes: a mother all in pink.

"Mom, she likes pink, the drawing is for her when she gets her leg fixed."

Yannick always finds excuses for the unexplained absences of his mother, who, as far as we know, is in good health, at least physically. But Yannick would certainly like his mother to be "fixed" forever.

At the start of the new school year, his mother had still not reappeared. Yannick was confronted with tales of their wonderful vacations by the other children, those with parents. So Yannick tells anyone who will listen about his own travels, his own beach, his visits to magnificent zoos with Mom.

It takes me a moment to realize that he's actually telling me about his real adventures with the real Lolo, whom he's named "Mom" in the fable of his imaginary vacation. I'm not sure what's blurred in the picture he's telling me, the identity of the mother or the reality of the events, or both.

As for the zoo, he dutifully puts the dinosaurs in jail.

The summer has dragged on, back-to-school is just a memory and Mum's absence from visits a bitter routine.

Yannick looks totally desperate: "Mum doesn't want to come anymore."

I try to put this terrible news into perspective: Mum is probably busy, she'll come another time, she's certainly thinking about him... Yannick doesn't listen to me. The grown-ups are constantly trying to reassure him of the love of this ever-absent mother, no doubt hoping to appease him. But these pious lies irritate his young teeth with the acid juice of the green grapes of well-intentioned but misleading words. He already knows the torment that will poison his existence: a fragile, fickle mother.

It's been several months now since his mother was released from prison, but she rarely shows up for the visits organized with her son. Yannick is back to his old self, the sweet, calm, affectionate little boy, perhaps a little more serious in his expressions.

Today, he looks pensive, serious, on the verge of sadness. He notices my "two big shy ones", two big teddy bears that have been lurking around, waiting for ages, each in his own armchair, to be addressed.

"Is this yours from when you were a kid?"

I stammer at this question, which catches me off guard... The next one too!

"Your mom and dad, are they in your house?"

How stupid grown-ups are! Stupidly, I reply that I've got white hair and that my mom and dad can't live in my house, since I've left theirs, as all children do one day... My answer seems to dismay him: he looks at me sidelong, frowning, slightly reproving.

Meditative, time-consuming, diligent and meticulous, he built a new, well-appointed prison with which he was very satisfied. He admires his work: "The prison is beautiful."

And suddenly, looking at me with a dark eye, he addresses me in a scathing tone:

"You can't leave home when you're grown up!"

Then, with a sad and resigned air:

"Where's Mom? Is she still in jail?"

Yannick is only three-and-a-half years old, and I'm amazed by his ability to sum up in two sentences all the tension in his life: his frustration at having such a fragile, absent mother, and his anguish at one day losing the emotional security provided by his foster family.

I noted in the margin of my file: "For Yannick, putting his mother in prison is a painful solution that allows him to 1 - keep her, i.e. insure himself against the risk of seeing her disappear 2 - be reassured that she has food and a place to sleep 3 - think that she can be cared for if necessary 4 - punish her for her abandonment."

Christmas approaches. Yannick explains that this time, his mother came to visit. She took him to the merry-go-round and they went for a hamburger.

"But she coughs," he adds.

It's the end of winter. Today, we played with a toy train, built a crazy circuit and played with dinosaurs. Yannick talked about making a prison, but then, caught up in the games, he forgot.

He told me absolutely nothing about his mother.

I didn't see Yannick again the following year. But not long ago, his mother was incarcerated again for several months. The anxiety, agitation and aggressiveness returned. Yannick demanded to see me again.

As soon as he entered my office, he rushed to the train track as if he'd left it the day before and declared:

"I want my mom to get out of prison, because she's my mom. My mommy is not the guards' mommy. My mommy, she's going to the judge and the judge is going to give me back my mommy."

Children always suffer from the fickleness of adults.

At the nursery, we see how depressed the little ones are when parents miss appointments and are repeatedly absent, each time with a new pretext that's even flimsier than the last. Admittedly, for some parents who haven't understood the meaning of the placement measure, it's heartbreaking to come and meet their child. But this avoidance shows that they feel their own suffering is more important than that of their child. However, this attitude of avoidance is better tolerated by social services than that of overly demanding parents, who are more difficult to deal with. Yet it is just as destructive. Out of respect for the child, no absence should be trivialized or ignored.

"What am I worth that neither Dad nor Mom deigns to even visit me, see my school, look at my report card, bring me a present on my birthday, inquire about what I do all day, how I'm growing up? I'm worthless. What's the point of making efforts to grow up if no one is there to pin them to the kitchen walls?"

But how many fathers and mothers of separated couples behave in this way towards their children when the ex has custody of them?

"My darling, hello, how are you? Well, I was supposed to pick you up this weekend, but something came up at the last minute, so I'll explain later. I hope you have

5. "Yannick Builds Prisons for Himself"

a good weekend. I'll be in touch. Well, put your mother on..."

"My little chick. My little cat. Did you have a good week? Your basketball game? Oh, is it this Sunday? The final? Of course I remembered!... You know, it's your father's weekend... Three o'clock! What a shame, I promised Roland I'd accompany him to an exhibition on the Neo-Impressionists. You know, Roland! I introduced you to him! The one with the art gallery. Come on! Come on, Roland! Don't get me wrong! It doesn't matter, there'll be other matches."

And what can we say about those parents who are never available - most of them fathers, but some mothers too - to accompany their child to a medical appointment, a teacher's appointment or a school outing? How proud the children are that both parents take time for them, and are sufficiently present at every stage of their development.

A childhood memory came back to me.

It was summer, and I must have been four or five years old. The sun was blazing down on a village square in the Spanish Cerdanya. An orchestra was playing in the bandstand under the plane trees. A few villagers were dancing. Suddenly, an imposing butcher stepped out from behind his stall, dropped his large knife, untied his stained apron and invited himself into the crowd. Then the grocer, or was it the baker, did the same. And then some more. I watched the stalls, the musicians and the sardana, waiting for the surprise of new dancers. And they did. Never in my childhood mind would I have imagined a butcher dancing with a grocer in a village square at midday. The miracle of music. The hypnotic fascination of a primitive folk scene.

Distracted for a moment from this rapture, I looked around. My parents were gone. I ran to look for them at random. Despite my age, I was acutely aware that I didn't know the language of this country, and that no one would understand me. I had lost my way in my thoughts and I had lost my parents.

How many little children wander around supermarkets like this until the call interrupts the insipid music: "A little brown girl, dressed in a blue sweater, is waiting for her mommy at reception." The mechanism is always the same. No longer able to see their mother or father, sometimes simply hidden by another shopper, children panic and set off blindly in search of their parents. The prevailing adultocentrism leads alarmed parents to say that their child is lost. But the child's reality is different. When a child gets lost, he doesn't say to himself "I'm lost", but "I've lost my parents".

For children whose parents fade away or are fickle, the feeling of doubt about their own worth is compounded by the worry of losing them. So they search for them in their heads, to the point where this imaginary journey sometimes invades the whole field of their thoughts.

Some, who have never known their father or mother due to early separation, divorce, placement or adoption, seem to have forgotten them. But it's not uncommon for them to take steps to find them when they reach adolescence or the age of majority. Sometimes much later.

"The train glides along with a pulsating metal beat. It's like giving birth in irons. I'm seventeen years, five months and nine days old. My father has been waiting for me for seventeen years, five months and nine days," writes Éric

5. "Yannick Builds Prisons for Himself"

Fottorino in *Questions à mon père*[22]. Day by day, he counts the time, which says a lot about a son's waiting.

If a parent thinks their child may have forgotten, they're wrong.

---

22. FOTTORINO (Éric), *Questions à mon père*, Paris, Gallimard, 2010.

6.
KARL DOESN'T KNOW WHAT TO DO WITH AN ADULT

Follow educational advice to the letter and you'll turn your child into an idiot.

ABALOURDI, "Child abalourdied by ill-treatment." *Littré*

Some situations are almost clinical conundrums, requiring us to reconstruct step by step the sequence of events that led a child to the nursery. Karl's is one such case.

We'd known Karl long before he was born. We had known his older sisters before him, and the children's judge had placed them in the service because they were in a state of near-abandonment, each showing significant emotional deficiencies. They were then placed in foster care. Little Stella had left us with the memory of a baby-specter who haunted the corridors while fleeing contact, a little ghost who remained glued to the sight of other children who wanted to play, cuddle and be with her. She never allowed herself to do the same, but she observed their activities keenly. If an adult approached her, even with infinite caution, she would withdraw like a knife from its shell. Necessity obliged us to take her in, feed her and care for her, but then she became absent, sinking into total passivity. It took months to tame her and watch her gradually build a personality.

When Karl's birth was announced, the professionals were convinced that the judge would order an early placement, since his parents were not investing in their children and were neglecting them. But no! The parents had made their mea culpa and amends, promises to follow all the advice, "yes yes" and "of course" to all the judge's demands and "judge, at last a boy, no more arguments, no more fights. We're back together, we're getting married, we're buying a house, we've got a job...".

The children's judge imposed regular educational supervision at home and psychological support in a care center. The parents were relatively compliant with these measures. On the days and at the times specified, Karl was taken into care and an educator visited his home every week. This arrangement seemed to reassure both the professionals and the judge.

We were still worried.

We met Karl's stroller when his mother deigned to visit her daughters. We knew the stroller, but not much about his face: his mother always kept him locked up under the hood. We had to let her know there was a baby inside, so she'd think about getting to know him a little. During a hearing at the judge's, the repeated remarks made in other circumstances came back to haunt her, and the mother moved to raise the stroller's hood. This left Karl with the sun in his eyes. He didn't even cry. An educator present was able to get the mother to move him away from the axis of the sun. In the dark or in the glare, Karl never flinched.

As time went by, the professionals who visited the child at home felt that Karl was well received, that he had a "good relationship" and that he was progressing - not very quickly, especially in terms of motor skills, but steadily. They even considered discontinuing the care, which became effective for four months due to poor administrative and judicial coordination. It was then that the older sister's revelations led to Karl's placement. With the parents in police custody for another matter, Karl was referred to the nursery at the age of two and a half, after four months without any professional visits.

Soon, consternation and anger rose up at the sight of this small, stunted child. He didn't speak, he didn't ask, he didn't cry. He seemed to fall asleep very late, alone in his bed, but he didn't call, didn't show, didn't protest. He didn't know how to hold himself in his carer's arms; he was so limp he would slip. You could catch him crying silently. Tears were the only thing to run down his impassive face. Often, his eyes would escape us.

The educators noted that he could walk, but like a diver. His head seemed too heavy to carry, bobbing at the end of his neck. He fell, banged himself, but didn't protect himself when he fell. No cries, no tears despite all the shocks, we felt for him, but he seemed insensitive and didn't seek consolation.

First enigma: on his arrival, despite this uncertain walk, he had no marks on his body. A few days later, the head of the department was surprised to find that he was covered in bruises from head to toe. Karl had discovered the freedom of walking and was falling a lot. But what about at home? Why had he arrived unmarked?

Second enigma: how could the professionals who knew and followed this child not have noticed the seriousness of his developmental delay and the construction of his personality? Worse still, the last professional team mandated by the judge to monitor the child at home concluded that the parents were progressing well and adhering to the educational work being done at home. Karl's developmental delay was attributed to "unexplained muscular weakness". He was therefore considered a deficient little boy, evolving at his own retarded pace.

To shed light on these mysteries, a meeting was organized with the various people who had followed this little boy since his birth.

Every week, Karl's mother took him to the psychological care center for a motor skills session, to compensate for his great delay in this area. She made trivial but appropriate remarks about her son's difficulties. Admittedly, she had refused the meetings with the psychologist on the flimsiest of pretexts, but she did ask for advice on exercises to be carried out at home between sessions.

The first of the judge's injunctions, assiduous follow-up of the child's care, had been respected.

A second observation from these professionals, who were working at home, and who, as good technicians respecting conventions in their approach to the parents, phoned them every time to agree their visiting schedule: the mother was always there to welcome them in a bright room, with her child in a bouncer or high chair and a few toys at hand. The judge's second injunction, to cooperate with the outpatient follow-up team, had also been respected. Better still, the mother also asked them for advice on feeding or bathing, questions that should have intrigued a mother of four.

A social worker from outside these first two teams, who had gone to meet the family unannounced to get documents signed, was astonished:

"When I came to the house, everything was closed, shutters, lights. It was late morning, and the house was pitch black. The living room was empty, with no toys. No Karl either, so I asked about him and his mother explained that he was asleep. At my insistence (a family once called me a social insister), she went to fetch him. He was still in his pyjamas, hadn't been changed, and I'm not sure if he'd been fed that morning. When I questioned her, her mother cut her short - 'We had friends over last night, we were up very late and so was Karl.' This struck me as suspicious, because I'd been there twice before to get them to sign papers, and all the shutters were closed, just as they were that morning. As no one had answered my doorbell, I had asked the neighbors about the presence of Karl's parents and they had told me that the house was always closed and that the shutters were rarely opened."

"But when we came," continued the educator, "the house was bright and the shutters were wide open. Karl was up and waiting, playing with toys. He was obviously happy to see us!"

The social worker continued:

"On another occasion, I came again for some papers, again in the late morning, shutters closed, madam wasn't there. Monsieur was asleep, so he got up and opened the door. 'Ha! My wife works, I was working last night.' And Karl? 'I don't know where he is. Maybe he's upstairs asleep.'

6. Karl Doesn't Know What to do with an Adult

Indeed, Karl was in his room, in the dark, not fed, not changed. When he saw me, he smiled."

Suddenly, the truth appears, terrible and dismaying.

The mother respected the judge's injunctions to the letter. Twice a week, at the appointed hour, Karl was on deck, prepared for the educators' visit or for his trip to the care center. It must have taken a great deal of effort for her to prepare him in this way, and it's not wrong for her to explain to the judge that she had done everything he'd demanded. But the rest of Karl's time was spent in bed, in the dark. The toys (which had remained surprisingly new) were not taken out of their crate until the day of the educator's visit. To demonstrate her willingness to accept these measures, she asked for advice on how to look after her son. To demonstrate her good will, she also asked a few questions about childcare, which the visitors, placed in a professional situation, were quick to answer. From time to time, she would pull Karl out of bed, like a green plant. Other observations would confirm this scenario.

Karl had become accustomed to not asking for anything, to total passivity. He could lie alone in bed for hours with his eyes open. Of course, he made little progress with his motor skills. There was no risk of him falling! The toys remained clean and new. And what a pleasure it was for this baby to find someone to look after him every week. And on this particular day, his mother miraculously became available.

The desert, sand dunes as far as the eye can see, dry heat, overwhelming light. I was lucky enough to bivouac there and discover the wonder of dawn. In the dawning light, well before the first rays, even before dawn, when the temperature is still bearable, a few rare grasses make the most of these precious moments, catching the moisture of a fine layer of mist: at this moment, their foliage is green. They're full of life in a matter of minutes. Invigorated by this thin, protective and beneficial veil, the desert is green! It's a rare, fleeting and moving moment that forever leaves its dewy stigma on the traveler's soul, as he marvels at the spectacle of life blossoming in the divinely opened gap between the frightening solitude of night and the deadly aridity of day. As soon as the sun comes out, the miracle evaporates and the grass turns to straw. But this was no mirage. Desert seeds know this, and can lie dormant for years, waiting for ideal conditions of temperature and humidity to germinate, grow and flower in a matter of days.

Karl was in a state of dormancy, passively awaiting the weekly arrival of these caravanners who allowed him to receive attention, light and words in a warm atmosphere, allowing him to exist for these short moments. By the simple regularity of their visits, without knowing it, they saved his life. Their absence of four months could have been fatal.

For a child, there is no worse mistreatment than neglect and oblivion.

There are some forgotten words that should be revived. *Abalourdi* is one of them. A long time ago, La Curne de Sainte-Palaye[23] stated: "This word still exists with a slight alteration in our word *abasourdir*", indicating that it had already fallen into disuse. Around 1690, La Furetière also considered its infinitive to have disappeared: "ABALOURDIR.

---

23. *Dictionnaire historique de l'ancien langage françois*, 1749.

6. Karl Doesn't Know What to do with an Adult

Vieux mot, et hors d'usage qui signifioit autrefois, 'abrutir, rendre stupide. estourdir."

Estourdir? Let's follow La Furetière's lead:

"Stun. To cause an emotion or derangement in the brain, or in the senses, which prevents them from doing their functions well."

Isn't that a luminous definition of anxious stupor? Furetière adds:

"ESTOURDIR, said figuratively in moral matters, of accidents that disturb, that surprise our reasons."

"Psychic trauma" was described by La Furetière more than two centuries before the psychiatric world defined it.

Not to be confused with :

"ESTOURBIR, v. tr. 19th century. To stun, to kill. *Fig.* To strike with stupor. He's still stunned by the news."

Very close to abasourdir. The Nouveau Dictionnaire de l'Académie tells us:

"ABASOURDIR, v. tr. 17th century. Derived from basourdir, "to kill" [...] *Fig.* To strike with stupor, to dismay. To overwhelm."

And *Littré*: "Stunned by an unforeseen misfortune."

Abasourdi: we're back to *abalourdir*, whose past participle was resurrected with surprising precision by the 19th-century *Littré*:

"ABALURDI, child abalurdi by mistreatment."

As a translator of Hippocrates and a keen observer of the infancy of modern medicine, had he read Ambroise Tardieu's forensic work on *Sévices et mauvais traitement exercés sur les enfants,* published in 1860? In any case, he introduced the clinical aspects of child psychiatry and maltreatment into our vocabulary. Yet it would take French society more than a century - until 1970 - to release doctors from professional secrecy and authorize them to report abused children to the courts.

And, paraphrasing Littré, it remains very topical to write:

"The child stunned by too much silence or unkind words, stunned by shouts or blows, if he doesn't end up simply stunned, is very likely to keep his mind stunned forever."

7.

Sophie: a Real Little Mother

When grown-ups are worse than children!

It was a bright morning, with the sun shining down on the cottage. Sophie got up early and decided to help her mother, who was still asleep. As the eldest of four children, she was already well-versed in running the household.

First of all, we had to take care of baby, who was starting to whimper, announcing the end of his sleep. But where could Mum have put the bottle? Sophie found the can of formula and asked:

"Baby, of, four, months, one hundred, four, twenties, grams of water, six, measures, of milk. Whoo! It's so complicated! Yes, it is! I can't squeeze the pacifier! Yes, you can! Shake well and I'll taste it. Mmm! It's so good! I'd like to give my little brother his bottle. But Mum won't let me, she says it's too expensive. Yes! Yes! I'm coming, I'm coming, your little mommy's coming, here's my baby! Ah, this cradle is too deep, Little Brother, help me so I can take you. You're so heavy! Well, I'll settle into the armchair.

Ah! Damn! I left the bottle on the table. I'll put you down and go and get it. Don't move or you'll fall out of the chair. Don't cry, you'll wake Mum! She's tired this morning, she must be sleeping! Come on, then! That's it! That's it! I'll take you back in the armchair and gloups! Drink your bottle. Not so fast! Not so fast! Your tummy's going to hurt again and you'll have to burp."

Between the carcasses of cans, the torn packaging of ready-made meals and the empty bottles strewn across the table, Sophie finds the telephone.

- Madam social worker, it's Sophie on the phone, are you all right? Did you sleep well? I'm glad to talk to you. Sometimes when I call, you're not there. They tell me you've taken your leave. Your mom and dad, are they ReTaiTés? Are you going to take them home for a walk? I don't think Mommy slept very well. She's still sleeping. She didn't take her ten camants yesterday. She didn't have enough. She said: "I'm not going to the chemist or I'll swallow it all." I think it was better that she didn't go. If she'd bought her ten pills, she'd have swallowed them all. Besides, she doesn't count her ten pills very well; sometimes she takes eleven or twelve.

- I know, Sophie, your mom takes way too many painkillers.

- There, she must have only eaten the bottom of the box. Because Mum lied to you when she said everything was fine. She sleeps on the couch all day and doesn't take care of her little brother. I'm the one who makes the bottles. Sometimes I do it with a spoon and then I taste it to see if it's good, sometimes I add water, sometimes milk. Because I don't like counting. On the milk can it's complicated. I like to dip my finger in the poude and lick it off my finger. Milk in poofs is good. It's all dry in the mouth afterwards. Mom doesn't want it, she says it's too expensive. When I put it in the bottle and some poude falls on the table, she scolds me. Once I ate some poo with a spoon, but I swallowed it all through the wrong hole. I coughed it up, spat it out, it was like snow flying, my brothers were laughing, it made me cough even more, I couldn't stop. They wanted some too, but I didn't give them any, they're too little, and then Mom would have yelled. But Mommy was asleep. Right now, Mommy's still asleep. That's why I'm calling you. I fed my little brother. I like giving him his bottle, he smiles a lot and tickles my cheek with his little hand. Then I woke up Bryan and Carlos. Bryan has wet the bed again, and it stinks. I gave them their cereal, but I washed the bowls because there weren't any clean ones left. Mom should go back to the hospital. She says if this keeps up, she'll throw herself out the window. If Mommy goes to the hospital, it's a shame, because I'll be going to a home and changing teachers again. The teacher's nice. She always asks how Mommy is. And then she always wants to know if I've eaten well, if my brothers are behaving, if the baby's okay, if Daddy's come, if he's been nice. The teacher always wants to know everything, but she's nice and I like her. I try to get good grades to please her. Maths is okay, but words are sometimes difficult, I don't really know the words. Mom didn't know what to call my little brother. So I chose the name. I was disappointed, I wanted to give him the teacher's name, Suzie, I think it's pretty, because I like the teacher. But Suzie is only suitable for girls. So I told Mom to call him Benji. It's better for a guy, and it's pretty too. In a TV movie, there was a dog named Benji. He was good with baby animals. Here, I'll give you Mommy. Mommy! Mommy! Mommy! Mommy! Wake up, it's the social worker on the phone.

7. Sophie: a Real Little Mother

- Ah! Madam assistant. Come quickly! I'm shaking all over, I want to die, I can't take care of the kids anymore. Come quickly!

- Madam social worker, when are you coming to pick us up to go to the shelter? Don't tell Dad. He hasn't been here for ages. If you tell Dad that Mum's going back to hospital, they'll argue and he'll come and beat her up. All the dads Mom's ever found drink alcohol and beat people up. Sometimes Mom drinks too. Sometimes it's Mum who beats him up when they go to the bar. I've packed school bags for Bryan and Carlos and a bag for the home with their cuddly toys. They don't sleep and they cry when they don't have their cuddly toys. But I couldn't find any snacks for school. Mom didn't do the shopping. I do them when I can find the money. Madam social worker, when are you coming? I really don't understand grown-ups.

And so, a few hours later, we received little Benji at the nursery, without Sophie who, for lack of space, was placed with a foster family.

Benji proved to be an alert baby, but he never wanted to be left alone or to leave his arms. He was quite difficult to reassure and calm. Rocking him in the arms, as if in a cradle, which babies like to do at this age, didn't satisfy him. His favorite position, the one that calmed him best, was to be carried upright against himself, straight and very high, almost balancing on his shoulder, which was rather curious.

Sophie had to wait over a week for a visit to be organized so that she could come and see her brothers on the ward.

As soon as she arrived at the nursery, Sophie discovered, undoubtedly alerted by the cries she had recognized, the educators entangled with this infant who was difficult to carry and calm. Her mother was carrying the child horizontally, with the baby's head resting on her left elbow, her small body supported by her hands, and her feet resting on her right elbow.

"He doesn't like to be held like that," she explained, "you have to take him under your arms, I'll show you."

And we were surprised to hear him add:

"Come on baby, come to Mommy."

And putting her money where her mouth was, she grabbed Petit-Frère, girdling him under her arms, and carried him like this, holding him facing her, while walking on her heels to maintain his balance. In this acrobatic position, with both arms gripping him tightly to prevent him from slipping, she was also unable to support her brother's small head, but the baby adapted, resting his head in his sister's neck. This strange crew, laden with too heavy a burden, began to jerk low, the little brother resting his head in his elder's collar, while the rest of his body dangled and swayed to the rhythm of this hectic dance. He calmed down instantly: Benji was used to this unusual carrying and rhythm. It was the technique Sophie had invented to cradle her little brother, handicapped as she was by being so slight and weighing no more than three times her own weight. It was then we realized that *she* had been his mother.

We stared at her, a little stunned, torn between admiration for so much skill for her age and dismay at the gravity of the burdens already weighing on her frail shoulders.

"Poor little mother," the nurse whispered to me, "she's just nine years old."

Sophie's story shows us how difficult it is to be a mother and pursue an education, have grown-up responsibilities and still be a carefree child. Sophie had a language delay, struggled at school and proved to be an anxious and complicated child. Her adolescence was extremely difficult, torn as she was between watching over and supporting her mother and feeling fed up with never having had the chance to be an innocent, serene child. From then on, she disastrously alternated back and forth between her foster family and her mother.

Normal" children often play the game of being their parents' parents. This reversal of roles helps to shape their image of family life. Prepare a dinner party for your parents. Announce that they'll travel the world, make their fortune and come back to fill them. Or that they'll own a big castle where they can welcome Mom or Dad. These fantasies of ambition and seduction are useful and necessary for a child's growth.

But these are just dreams and games.

It's an unbearable burden for a child to have to exist alone. If his parents fail, he will exhaust himself supporting them, whatever the cost. By the end of his life, in 1932, Ferenczi had masterfully described this parentification[24] of the child in an original text[25], in which he wrote, among other things: "A mother who continually complains about her suffering can transform her child into a caregiver, that is to say, into a veritable maternal substitute, without

---

24. Several other neologisms are used to describe this state: *adulto-morphism, hyper-maturation, parentified child*, etc.

25. FERENCZI (Sandor), "Confusion de langue entre les adultes et l'enfant", 1932, in *Psychanalyse. Œuvres complètes. Tome IV (1927-1933)*, Paris, Payot, 1982, p. 225.

taking into account the child's own interests." Children who are forced to inhabit this inverted role between adult and child are found in situations of severe parental weakness, sometimes due to illness, depression, mental disorder or alcoholism.

Another form of parentification is found in very ill children. These children perceive the severity of their condition through their parents' distress. Realizing that they are in vital danger and that their parents cannot endure it, they sometimes have no other recourse than to support them through this ordeal. This artifice gives them the illusion of not having to bear both their parents' distress and their own loneliness. To be the prop of one's own support: an impossible task.

This role reversal is also found in another configuration: that of the so-called little geniuses, athletes or intellectually gifted children whose parents push them to extremes. These parents, with their sickly narcissism, vampire and feast on the supposedly exceptional talents of their offspring to the point of reducing them to sterile beings, withered too soon. What a waste! True geniuses are rare, exceptional and free themselves from adults in order to blossom.

Early success comes at a cost. The benefits that parents delude themselves into receiving from the pride of having such a remarkable offspring, will have to be paid for by the child, at a high price. Because of their physical, psychological and emotional dependence, children always feel indebted to their parents. There's no need to imagine the folly of adding to the bill.

No doubt these parents should reread Plutarch, who wrote twenty centuries ago: "Another thing: I've seen some fathers who, by dint of loving their children, had come to

7. Sophie: a Real Little Mother

love them not at all. What do I mean by saying this? An example will make my point clearer. In their ardent desire to see their sons quickly become the first in everything, they impose on them a workload that has no proportion, under which they succumb discouraged; and moreover, overwhelmed by the excess of fatigue, they no longer receive instruction with docility. Well, just as plants thrive if watered moderately, but too much water suffocates them, so the mind grows through measured study, but is drowned by excessive work. Children must therefore be allowed to catch their breath, far from occupying them relentlessly."[26]

26. PLUTARCH, 1st century AD (*Œuvres morales, Sur l'éducation des enfants*: œuvre complète), chapter XIII.

8.

THE ENIGMA OF ARRIVAL

With your child, you'll always be off the mark!

A tribute to V.S. Naipaul

"What is it like to have a baby? No matter how much I prepared myself for those first moments, the stress overwhelmed everything! My mind was running on empty. It reminded me of the time of waiting before meeting my own children, when they were born. Oddly enough, it remained associated in my memory with the artificial scents of cleaning products, the impeccable linoleum running up the baseboard, the impersonal pastels on the walls, those silly details that capture your mind when you're waiting your turn at a crossroads of destiny. Then came the surprise of the meeting and the soft luminosity of the room, which matched the pride and joy of those precious moments. And then the emotional contemplation of this new child.

But for this child I was about to meet, the unknown was much stronger. He was a child who already had his own story. He was a child who had suffered. It was also the discovery of the demands of teamwork and new responsibilities for which I would be accountable.

I was suddenly very tense when the educator went to pick him up. It was hard for me to imagine him, as this was his first experience. I'd seen photos of him, his heavy head tilted, his eyes looking down, giving him a very sad look. Was it sadness, in fact? What was I going to do to tame him? All these questions flew by, but I also knew that reality was bound to turn everything upside down and make a place for itself."

At the team meeting, we go over the story of three-year-old Karl's first meeting with Alain, a brand-new "childminder". Alain has embarked on this new adventure after a lifetime's work. His children are grown up, but this is a first for him, and for Karl too.

At the nursery, we always take great care to carefully analyze the initial moments when a child meets his or her caregiver, as well as the evolution of their relationship in the first few months. Children with attachment disorders have difficulty creating and sustaining emotional bonds. Their apparent indifference, their sometimes spectacular insecurity, even their opposition, can worry the caregiver to the point of making him/her think that the child is refusing him/her. This initial misunderstanding can be fatal for the rest of the placement. With children who are so unable to bond, short-term placement failures are not uncommon, with foster carers sometimes giving up after a few weeks or months. It's to try and avoid these devastating misunderstandings that we've introduced this meticulous monitoring system.

To help us understand the child's difficulty in establishing a secure emotional relationship after a disastrous and destructive experience with his parents, I like to tell new family assistants the story of "Dylan at the campsite".

After two years in the nursery, Dylan, who had arrived in a state of psychological stress, went to live with a foster family where he quickly found his bearings and adapted wonderfully. He very quickly put his trust in his foster carer, whom he follows everywhere and never wants to leave. His only little quirk is that he has difficulty going out alone in front of the house. Dylan doesn't like to play on the nearby terrace or lawn. If a noise or unusual event, however small, disturbs his environment, he returns belly-down to take refuge inside the house or in his foster mother's petticoats. A plane high in the sky, its rumble barely audible, and our Dylan scurries back into the house. A dog barking a few houses away, same effect. But apart from that, everything seems to be going well: Dylan is smiling, playful, active, talkative, eats well, sleeps well and is making progress every day. A year after his arrival in this family, his nursery assistant was delighted to take him "camping" to introduce him to the pleasures of the seaside, the beach and the sand. An almost initiatory step in the education of today's children. Discovering the sea, that shifting space where the boundaries between ocean, land and sky are neither clear nor blurred, but always changing, constantly redrawn by the wind, clouds, sun and moon. Powerful, powerful sensory emotions, in tune with the elements. A two-week vacation is bliss! Dylan joins in by mimicry, but without any real conviction, the light exaltation that presides over this departure.

The first night at the campsite is a disaster: Dylan cries and can't leave his nanny's arms. The day is no easier. The days and nights that followed were no different. Exhaustion set in, and the hoped-for joy of the vacation fizzled out. In desperation, the family decides to shorten the stay. Dylan is told that in two days, we'll be heading home. Dylan had heard the words "going home" and the effect was magical: he slept like a log for the last two nights, and was extraordinarily happy to find his home again. He had probably imagined that this vacation was a journey of no return. What he hadn't realized was that this stay away from home was temporary. It was his "home" that had allowed him to discover emotional security. The next vacation... went well... What's even funnier is that this story coincided with the release of Spielberg's *E.T.*, in which the little extraterrestrial tirelessly repeats "home phone".

On arrival at the nursery, some babies or young children, because of the traumatic life they have lived before, are sometimes so insecure that even changing rooms can worry them. In some cases, it takes them several weeks to agree to visit the corridors of the establishment. And then only gradually, with a very precise security perimeter. Going outside is no easy matter. The reality of these children's major insecurity seems incomprehensible to some professionals who are discovering this world apart, where the usual benchmarks for childhood are inoperative. One of our young directors, fresh out of director's school and with his mouth full of books on the education of children - the normal ones, of course, the ones who know how to adapt - had tried mordicus to move the doctor's surgery to distant buildings, chanting that in normal life, children go to the doctor outside the house and not the other way round. An unfortunate attempt to show off her knowledge, impose her authority on the professionals and try to normalize our little boarders by coercion. It's hard to get her to understand that, for some traumatized children, the simple act of leaving their living quarters to cross the hallway can provoke insane insecurity, or that getting into a car to leave the home can sometimes cause real panic.

Back to Karl. Alain continues:

"And then I heard the educator and Karl's footsteps in the corridor. The door had been left ajar. I can't see them, but I can hear her talking to Karl. My heart is pounding, but I've seen it all before, and I want to stay calm and cool. Karl suddenly appears in the doorway. He's standing there all alone. He steps forward to enter. We're face to face. He doesn't look at me. I can't see his face. He hasn't entered the room. He said 'no'. He turned on his heel and disappeared. It all happened so fast, the educator didn't even have time to catch up with him.

I was shocked, sorry, disappointed and worried. What's more, the educator started laughing. She seemed amused by the child's reaction. She was even delighted. She explained that this was real progress, one of the first times Karl had used the 'no' and allowed himself to show his emotions. She was very happy about this progress in Karl, who was about to turn three. But I wasn't happy about it, I was crushed.

The educator was satisfied. The solemnity of the event and the emotional charge of the meeting had undoubtedly enabled Karl to have this reaction, which she considered positive. But with this refusal, I felt a break within me. I had imagined that the child would agree. I had imagined a child who would wait for me, but he told me 'no', head-on.

In the car, on the way home, the story of that first meeting flashed before my eyes. Karl came forward, but didn't enter the room. We were face to face. He didn't look at me. He said 'no', turned on his heel and disappeared. What's more, the teacher started laughing. What followed was just as disappointing as the initial fiasco.

Karl had escaped, so the educator came back with him, holding his hand, and introduced me: 'Karl, this is Alain, you're going to live with him.' Karl didn't look at me, but a little later, he hit his sternum with his little fist, belching out a very guttural 'Karl'. Then he took refuge in the dinette corner to hide, and the approach was complicated. In the end, however, he gave me furtive glances. I caught a glimpse of his dark beads from underneath. Then he accepted my presence, quite close to him, while he explored the toy box. I'd brought him a small stuffed toy as a gift. He refused it. The educator tried to comfort me, telling me she'd put my welcome gift in his room. A magnificent consolation prize. My cuddly toy on his shelf!

I couldn't understand why the educator maintained her calm, confident attitude. Nothing was working, but she remained serene and seemed to be enjoying the situation. I wasn't! The collapse. I said to myself, 'That's it, the team is going to offer me another child!'

The following night, I watched the film again. Usually, the night clouds the judgment, but here, other elements come back to me, more encouraging.

Karl stood by the dinette. He remained aloof, but in a detail I hadn't noticed, he kept under his arm the small photo album of our family that I had brought to the educators before this meeting so that they could tell him about me and the household. They told me he refused to look at it. But today, at that meeting, he was holding it tightly. Incidentally, I understood much later that the photos and the contents of the album were of little use, as he wasn't at all interested in the images. But he kept the album as an object that came from me. He had refused my stuffed toy, but he treasured the object-album handed to him two days earlier by the educators. Then I also remembered that, while he had run away, he had later stealthily leaned his back against me as he rummaged through the toy box. This prolonged leaning proved that it wasn't accidental.

Suddenly, I understood the enormous effort Karl had made to come and meet me, even though he didn't know me. We were strangers to each other, but our destinies were bound to cross for a while. I thought I had to tame him, but my approaches were in vain. I asked him to come and meet me, to accept my cuddly toy, to read my photo album, to look at me. He refused to accept my stuffed toy, to read my photo album, to run away from me and to look at me.

But Karl had sent me messages I hadn't noticed because they weren't the ones I'd imagined I'd receive. In reality, it was he who had come to me, and I had seen nothing.

He showed me how attached he was to coming to my family by holding our photo album close to him. He introduced himself to me by calling himself 'Karl', which he pronounced in a guttural tone, and pointed to himself with a fist to the chest. He leaned against me for a moment and willingly met my gaze for a few moments, glancing at me from underneath the photos. I thought I had to tame him, but he'd chosen me. It was hard to decipher. He'd say 'no', but he'd say 'yes'. Since then, I've learned to decipher these paradoxes.

It was at this point that I also realized how much it meant to him to have to leave the educators he had become so attached to. Despite this sacrifice, he had come to me.

Full of hope, I looked forward to the second meeting with real impatience."

Meeting a child is always unpredictable. And understanding them is full of surprises.

A child is a novelty.

Locke[27], an English philosopher, published a series of texts on education in 1693, in which he spoke out against child abuse. He concluded his work by revealing his conception of the child as a being to be molded. "I only wanted to set out a few general views here, which relate to the main aim of education. They were, moreover, intended for the son of a gentleman friend of mine, whom I considered, because of his young age, as a blank page or a piece of wax that I could shape and mold to my liking."

This unpublished Locke is a child that the adult must write.

No, it's not! The child I'm talking about is an unpublished version of himself.

There are now more than seven billion old babies on this earth. More than a hundred billion others have preceded us. Billions and billions of different emotions and thoughts.

But a baby's means of expression - crying and laughing, silences and cries, smiles and sulks, oppositional attitudes and tender gestures, bodily aches and pains and pleasures of life - remain very limited in number. A child who cries

---

27. LOCKE, *Quelques pensées sur l'éducation*, (1693), translated from English by G. Compayré, Paris, Hachette, 1909.

the moment he is separated from his mother does not indicate whether he is mourning for her, worried about her, not being well looked after by his nanny, has a toothache or is simply tired. For older children, their access to speech does not guarantee that they will imagine or consider it possible to express their torment. Children also have their pride, their self-importance and their concern not to burden their parents with their problems.

No expression, no manifestation of a child is specific to anything. Any behavior can mean a thousand things. Parents often interpret a change in their child's behavior in a precise, univocal sense, leading to misunderstanding and confusion.

Not only does the child not feel heard in the way he expresses himself, but his feelings and concerns are crushed by the adult who claims to know for him. The paradigm of this impasse is the slap that silences the child, accompanied by "why are you crying? don't you know? well, now you will!"

9.
SIMON CRIES OUT FOR LIFE AND DEATH

Saying no to violence

"I'd never have thought it possible to have a four-month-old baby mistreated. The pediatrician had given me a very gloomy description of him, the bruises on his face, the black eyes, his insecurity, his difficulty feeding himself. The educators had described him as a wild kitten, uttering little plaintive, haunting cries, panicking as soon as anyone got near.

We were first introduced to each other when he was seven months old. Obviously, I reassured myself that, three months after the event, I wouldn't have to see his swollen face. And yet, I was shocked by this encounter. I'll always remember those first moments. His complexion was haggard, almost gray, his face hollow and disharmonious, his face a frightening little old man, his hair poor and dry. He wasn't handsome... I can't say he was ugly. He smiled blankly, without address, offering nothing gratifying to his touch. I couldn't meet his eyes, so much so that I wondered, just for a few seconds, if I'd ever get attached to this child. I think I can even say that at the time, I felt a sense of dread... Which I didn't admit and understand until much later... You don't admit that sort of thing to yourself easily. It was a baby! I was welcoming a new child! I had to be positive!

Service meeting. Esther, the nursery's new childminder, tells us about her first meeting with Simon. Her naiveté in the profession, in the noble sense of the word, still leaves her with the capacity to be astonished and moved. And the apt description she offers is reminiscent of many of the other babies we take in. When they are first admitted, they often have the crumpled face of a little old man, a haggard complexion, dry hair, an inexpressive or evasive expression, clenched fists and a stiff body. Scary babies.

The rest of this first meeting with Esther had gone rather smoothly. Annie, his educator, gently placed Simon in Esther's arms. Simon's body was hard and very stiff. But he relaxed and curled up against her. Then he began to suckle her silk scarf. Then he'd agreed to eat.

But their eyes didn't meet.

Only then did he stare at Esther. With a piercing gaze of insane acuity. It was as if he'd had her scanned. You never see that in a baby's eyes. A gaze that probes and pierces at the same time. A look that clings to you and tears at your heart, imploring and violent. It was a gaze that was hard to bear, and it unsettled Esther. Annie had first reassured Simon:

"You're in Esther's arms. You'll go to her soon."

Annie then spoke to Esther about Simon, to give her renewed confidence. After three months in the nursery, Simon was having difficulty adapting to the rhythm of the structure and was eating very poorly - a child who showed no appetite for life - his evolution was worrying and the team had decided to entrust him to a foster family. When Esther was approached, Annie spoke to Simon about her. He probably didn't understand everything, but he sensed the concern the educators had for him. From that day on, he began to eat a little more properly. He had been waiting for this moment! He was already feeling better!

Simon left a few days later for Esther's house.

And at Esther's, all hell broke loose!

Those unfamiliar with abused babies think it's easy to look after an infant, because it's small, sleeps, eats and doesn't make much noise. But think again! A suffering baby can just as easily blow up a team of seasoned professionals in a nursery or an experienced foster family as a sick, violent and destructive teenager ransacking a home or institution. The screams and cries of these children, their sleep disturbances - seeing a baby sleep with his eyes open is terrifying - or their refusal to eat - they each have their own particularity - generate unbearable anguish. With the feeling that there's nothing we can do for them, and no way of relieving them.

A baby can writhe in psychic pain. And since this psychic pain is linked to his inability to trust the adult, he feels himself falling endlessly, even if he's in your arms. As Homer tells Hephaestus, a baby thrown down from Olympus by his mother: "All day long I fell, and at sunset I fell to Lemnos, having but one breath of life left. Suffering came to me, after the long fall willed by my bitch-eyed mother, who wished to hide me, because I was lame."[28]

-----

28. HOMER, *Iliad*, Canto XVIII, translation by Itinera Electronica, Université catholique de Louvain.

Ah! of course, Simon ate better and gained weight, which meant he was doing better, the pediatrician would be satisfied, but it was the horror! Day and night. Especially at night!

Simon exuded stress and fear, something impossible to contain. He was always on the alert, on the lookout, like a hunted beast. Esther went down into the underworld with him. And Simon showed her everything.

He was terrified as soon as the noise level increased. He instantly regained his piercing, scrutinizing gaze. If one of Esther's children sang, laughed or spoke a little loudly, Simon would stiffen that very second. A loud noise and he would jump as if he'd received an electric shock. Esther learned to reassure him: "Don't worry, laughter is not dangerous! Exploding joy does no harm! The lively voice that crackles doesn't hurt!"

Soon enough, he was using Esther to gauge the environment and assess whether the situation was dangerous, harmless or friendly. Simon would look for her with his eyes to interpret the tone of the atmosphere and know where he stood. During the day, Esther's presence seemed to be enough to calm his nerves.

But at night, it was frightening. As soon as evening arrived, the haunting cry of a plaintive kitten would creep into every room of the house, conveying a dark, heavy atmosphere. Esther's house seemed haunted. The mournful, goosebump-inducing cry intensified as soon as a ray of light entered her room. At this point, Simon panicked completely. If Esther picked him up to soothe him, he'd throw his head back and stare at the lamp, screaming even louder, to burst his eardrums. Hoarse, heart-stopping screams that grabbed you by the gut. It was unthinkable to leave him crying in his crib with the wail of a skinned little animal. It was equally impossible to soothe and reassure him, as any attempt to do so would only aggravate his cries and terror.

Esther tells us:

"I saw the scene. Those hoarse, throbbing cries, exasperated screams in response, the light coming on, the blows falling. This child's cries were putting him in danger at his parents' house. It was at night that he had to be beaten. One night, I was so tired - it had been going on for two months - and his cries were so loud that I thought of locking him in the garage. Not to punish him - do you punish a nine-month-old? No, to stop hearing him. I didn't want to hear it anymore. He was reaching a limit with me, it was getting violent, I felt attacked, I was at my wits' end, I was very scared. That's when I saw what had happened...

So I said to him - in the middle of his cries - I said 'I won't hurt you, I don't know what to do, but I won't hurt you'. I took him in his crib - he was crying - I told him 'I won't hit you', he calmed down a little - he was a little cold, he was wet -, I changed him, dried him, wrapped him up, held him against me. He stayed calm, and it was from that night on that he calmed down. He had wanted me to hear, he had wanted to show me."

I recapitulate the case, the circumstances. When the density of experience is too great, immersing yourself in concrete, palpable objects - administrative paperwork, court orders, medical certificates - gives you a sense of contentment.

A mother with nothing to live for: poor, abused, swindled, racketeered, her apartment squatted. She herself has been made homeless by her attackers, who occupy the

9. Simon Cries Out for Life and Death

premises in her place. They were acquaintances, including Simon's father, a violent man incarcerated several times for this reason. The sordid, the real, the strong. Pitiful trafficking and petty theft of all kinds, police raids. Emotional, intellectual and cultural poverty oozes from the file, dripping from the documents. Despite the convoluted and convoluted judicial language, you can see the cockroaches that run between the pages, from which emanates a misery that stinks and grabs you by the throat. Simon's mother, unable to defend herself, takes the rap for the others. Women's prison. Simon is born. Who's the father? Domestic violence. Simon in hospital... bruises... parents' stupidity and incoherence. How did it happen? Well, he did it to himself - Simon is only four months old! -placement by the public prosecutor.

A mother unable to protect herself from others, let alone reassure, contain and soothe a baby. She herself is terrified of the father, but can't do without him. Mother terrified of this crying baby, what to do, what to do, what to do. A vicious circle of mutual anxiety and fear. The more the baby cries, the less she knows what to do. The less she can reassure him, the more he cries. A concentration of anxiety between him and her. No meetings, just pile-ups. Never thought she could ask for advice or help. Just imagine changing a baby in these conditions, washing his hair, cutting his nails or blowing his nose. He doesn't even want a bottle. The crying, the screaming, the anxiety. How do you deal with him? Keep him quiet.

Now, a few months later, during visits, she seems extremely proud to be the mother of this child, eating him with her eyes. But she approaches him awkwardly, rushes to embrace him and devours him with kisses. But as soon as she steps forward, Simon starts whimpering. She panics, backs off and immediately asks the caregivers to take care of him for her. Her few questions are totally out of tune with the child's reality. Shortly after Easter - Simon is less than a year old and not yet able to stand up - she asks if he's been out looking for eggs in the garden... She's incapable of making any kind of assessment of Simon's progress. She has a son, and that's enough for her. His needs, his difficulties, his delays, his mistreatment - nothing intrigues her, nothing disturbs her. But Simon's whining terrorizes her.

Esther continues:
"Why didn't I lose it? Yet Simon dragged me into this spiral of violence and anguish. A child screaming like that is the ultimate alarm. A child who screams like that transmits absolute distress, vital anguish, and if you can't calm him down, the perception of your own powerlessness becomes absolutely unbearable, even threatening. If some people commit suicide because they no longer want to suffer the pain of living, perhaps some parents may come to the point of striking to stop hearing a child cry."

As Esther speaks, images come to mind. Reminiscences of readings and films invade me.

Maybe it's a story about an ethnic massacre in Bosnia or Rwanda, a Gestapo raid in a Jewish neighborhood. A woman with her baby, hidden in a makeshift cache. She hears predators approaching, the clatter of weapons or the crunch of whetstone on machete edges. Her heart wants to explode and hurts, she holds her breath and her movements, but is overwhelmed by wave after wave of tremors that jolt through her. She feels frozen. The cold steel of fate's scythe has already entered her.

9. Simon Cries Out for Life and Death

The baby senses from his mother's reaction that danger threatens. He wrinkles his forehead, stares at her and the tip of his chin begins to quiver. His mother, doubly distraught - the vital danger on the one hand, the risk of her son crying on the other - panics. But in a superhuman move, in an act of prodigious faith in her child, she suddenly overcomes her panic. She ignores the vital danger. She concentrates solely on the child. She tries to capture the baby's attention, to give him a change of scene. Reassure him first, and maybe they'll be saved. Overcome her terror to calm the baby. Before the first sob betrays them, she smiles at him, amuses him with comical little grimaces, the kind he loves, and strokes his cheek and neck with a finger. She hears footsteps approaching and her heart races. With measured gestures, controlling her ever-threatening tremors, she offers him her breast. Her son plunges his eyes into hers, they are alone in the world. He calms down, he won't cry, no sound will betray them. The men move away. They are saved. All she hears is a discreet little rhythmic sucking sound and her heart pounding, pounding. The baby watches in amazement as tears of relief glisten on her mother's smile.

"You're the sweetest baby, you saved us."

At the dawn of humanity, man became an increasingly dangerous predator for his environment and his fellow creatures, while our prehistoric ancestors must have known the terror of the great beasts and the constant fear of aggression that still haunts children's nightmares.

A child who cries and does not calm down quickly with appropriate care awakens in us ancestral and archaic fears, the fear of revealing the baby's presence and our own to predators and enemies[29].

Coincidentally, through the open French window - the nursery occupies the wooded grounds of a former convent - I hear the shrill warning call of a blackbird. Soon I catch a glimpse of it flying low over the lawn, mimicking a flapping wing, pursued by a naïve young cat that's falling for this game of decoy. As soon as the feline approaches, the bird regains its ease and, with a short flight, maintains a safe distance. The brood probably left the nest this morning, and woe betide anyone who doesn't hear the warning signal, keeps quiet and waits for this pseudo-sacrifice by their parent, which is not without risk, to keep the tiger away from the gardens.

No chromosome, no gene, no instinct has programmed humankind to protect its young. When prehistoric man, a nomadic hunter, became a sedentary shepherd, children, who until then could be an adjustment variable for the group - infanticide is structural to the history of mankind, to the history of our humanity - became arms and an economic force useful to the community. The child's status then changed profoundly. The child became precious. This new place for the child has overturned human beliefs and ideologies. This "new child" subverted the previous self- and world-views of the parents, who became parents - "new parents" in the modern sense of the word. But every human being, every child, every parent,

---

29. "I had a nightmare," says eight-year-old Julien, "in a room where I sleep with my sister, and there's a wolf. If you make a gesture, if you speak, if you make a noise, if you make a single body movement, the wolf wakes up and devours you."

9. Simon Cries Out for Life and Death

must retrace this path of refusal, and must be marked by the taboo of violence and infanticide. This psychic mark comes to us from the time when man changed his life, settled on a piece of land, cultivated it and built tombs for his ancestors and villages for his children. Today, these millennia-old foundations of humanity are shifting and shaking the family: man has left the land to live in cities[30], but that's another story.

While early-onset abuse such as Simon's is not common, it is by no means exceptional. More often than not, they are the result of parents with serious personality disorders. Hitting a baby is a sign of mental pathology, or of dramatic defects in self-construction.

The many recent cases of frozen babies[31] have only served to remind the media of a recurring fact: infanticide has always existed and continues to do so in our societies. But everyone wants to ignore it. Recent research by Dr Anne Tursz and her team at Inserm (France's National Institute for Health and Medical Research)[32] shows that the number of cases of infanticide in children under one year of age is grossly underestimated. In France, there are several dozen cases a year, or even hundreds, depending on the method of calculation. In the USA, homicide is considered the leading cause of traumatic death in children under one year of age. Reasoning on the principle of disaster medicine or road accident counts

---

30. In 2011, 50% of humanity lived in cities. Demographers estimate that this figure will rise to 60% before 2030.

31. Pithiviers 2000, Tours 2006, Albertville 2007, Guingamp 2008, Lasbordes 2011.

32. Tursz (Anne), *Les Oubliés. Enfants maltraités en France et par la France*, Paris, Éditions du Seuil, March 2010.

- for every death recorded, there are ten injuries - we can consider that early maltreatment is probably ten times more numerous, and therefore greatly underestimated in France.

Some exasperated parents, lacking in protective care, may also resort to shaking a crying baby to silence him or her, which is extremely dangerous. This is also serious abuse.

One mother told me about a scene she had witnessed one evening on her way home from work. Her husband was babysitting her four-month-old daughter. Exasperated by the child's crying, he took her under his arms, lifted her up to his face and started shaking her like a shaker, shouting at her to be quiet. "Suddenly, her little head knocked on his shoulder, then fell forward against his chest. She stopped screaming. I said to my husband, 'What have you done? She won't move! She's all limp! Has she lost consciousness?' He replied: 'It's not serious, the last time she woke up very quickly and then she slept. That way, she didn't cry anymore.'"

Foolishness knows no bounds.

Babies who can't hold their heads yet need to be handled with care, because of their muscular weakness. Shaking a baby can simply kill it, or disable it for life by causing irreversible brain damage. We've had several such babies in our nursery, some of them very disabled. It is estimated that there are at least two hundred cases of shaken babies every year in France... perhaps many more.

Simultaneous hemorrhages of the brain and retina, characteristic of such trauma, have been described in infants since the early 20th century. At the time, the cause was unknown. And it was not until 1972 that an American pediatrician and radiologist, John Caffey[33], attributed them to the consequences of violent shaking of the child...

But some parents are just as helpless with older children.

It's not uncommon for me to hear quite ordinary parents say: "I came for a consultation because the other day I thought I was going to lose it and hit him. It's been difficult for a while, but now I can't take it anymore. He's pushing me to the limit. We've got to do something to make it stop."

Or: "I have to tell you that I slapped her in the face for the first time. She had two bruised fingers on her cheek. I didn't sleep all night. I apologized, but I don't want it to happen again. What can I do?"

And again: "I couldn't find any other way to calm him down than to put him fully clothed under a cold shower. But I think that's barbaric!"

There's a fundamental difference between those parents who once made an impulsive, limited gesture and then regretted it, and those who institute physical sanctions as the usual educational standard or as a desperate solution to enforce their failing authority.

The former will most often call on their doctor, a psychologist or a child psychiatrist to find solutions to their educational difficulties. They can also seek help on a contractual basis from social services or the PMI.

---

33. It was John Caffey who first described the radiological syndrome of battered children in 1946. At the time, no one wanted to give credence to his work. It took almost twenty years for the scientific community to recognize these descriptions. This is a good example of the continuing social denial of the reality of child abuse. In 1860, Tardieu, a French forensic pathologist, experienced the same hostility and disbelief from his colleagues following the publication of his book *Mauvais traitements et sévices exercés sur les enfants*.

The latter, who fail to appreciate the seriousness of their actions, are subject to compulsory social or legal care, or even the removal of their children if home help measures prove insufficient.

Violence is not only useless, but above all toxic in the education of children. Masked as an assertion of authority, it's an admission of confusion and powerlessness.

Our family law is still rooted in the law of Roman antiquity, itself inspired by the law of Greek antiquity. For the Romans, the hand was the symbol of authority and strength, and in law, the *manus* signified the "power of the *pater familias*". This legal term of *manus*[34] succeeded the term *vis* - from which we derive the word *violence* - or the right to recover one's property by force. There was thus a direct relationship between authority and violence from the very beginnings of Greek and Roman law, which is no doubt not unrelated to the constant confusion that has persisted between authority and violence for centuries. The contemporary debate on the right of parents to correct their children, which took place at the Council of Europe in April 2010[35], is a reminder of this.

But what is authority?
It's the right to say no. It's not the right to be violent.

---

34. DAREMBERG and SAGLIO, *Dictionnaire des Antiquités grecques et romaines,* in ten volumes published between 1877 and 1919.

35. "Thirty years after Sweden banned corporal punishment, opponents of child abuse are organizing a debate under the aegis of the Council of Europe in Strasbourg on Tuesday, April 27, 2010 [...] The forty-seven member states want to launch a major 'Raise your hand against spanking' campaign", *Le Monde,* April 27, 2010.

9. Simon Cries Out for Life and Death

It's around eighteen months, two years, that the child understands the full meaning of "no" when he or she tries to experience its force. This does not mean, however, that they are not capable of hearing this "no", as early as their second year.

To say "no" is to deprive, to impose a sacrifice. Children who, at the age of two, are in the process of asserting themselves, a brand-new self whose clothes and stripes they want to wear for the first time, also want to be loved. In other words, to have their emotional needs met. Parents' first instinct is to rush to provide for them. It feels so good to respond to the needs of a child, of one's child.

But to say "no" is first to make a deprivation of oneself, to impose a sacrifice on oneself, respecting one's own ethics, before imposing it on the child.

"No! You've eaten enough, even though I'm so proud that you like my pancakes so much."

"No! I've already read you two stories and that's enough, now I want to be with your mother."

"No! You can't sleep in Mum and Dad's bed, it's our love bed. If one day you're sick, we can put a little extra bed in our room if you need it. But not our bed!"

On this subject, I can't resist recalling Freud's account of the educational conflict between the parents of little Hans[36], concerning the phobic boy's habit of coming to his mother's bed every morning. In one of his letters to Freud, the father writes: "A scene has played out every morning these past few days. Hans comes to us early every morning, and my wife *can't resist* taking him to bed for a few minutes.

---

36. "Le petit Hans", in *Cinq psychanalyses*, Paris, PUF, 1981, 10th edition.

I always start by telling her that she shouldn't take him to bed like that, and she sometimes replies, *rather excitedly*[37], that it's nonsense, that one minute can't do anything, and so on. Hans then stays with her for a little while." But it's a triumphant Hans whose imposture, permitted by his mother and unchallenged by his father, constitutes a taking of possession of the mother, "a fantasy of defiance linked to the satisfaction of having triumphed over paternal resistance. "Scream all you want, Mommy will still take me to bed and Mommy belongs to me!", adds Freud.

If parents are capable of consistently and correctly refusing to do anything with their child, out of playfulness, pleasure, weakness or weariness, by not changing domestic laws every day, the child soon understands that authority is not a whim, but a protection. And that Mum's or Dad's word is not just an empty word. It's not a radio you turn on when you feel like listening, and turn off when you don't feel like it anymore. It's a true and constant word. Which is very reassuring.

Imagine for a moment that the rules of the road changed from one day to the next, that the direction of traffic was random and that you didn't know in the morning whether cars were driving on the sidewalk or on the road that day. It would be too dangerous to leave your house. Conventions and laws, which are contractual, reassure, protect and regulate living together.

---

37. In a first translation of the text, Marie Bonaparte had translated "assez irritée" ("quite irritated"). Lacan, in *Le Séminaire*, Book IV, "La relation d'objet", corrects this error and translates "tout excitée", which speaks volumes about Hans' mother's difficulty in renouncing her own jouissance vis-à-vis her son. The words are underlined by the author of the present work.

9. Simon Cries Out for Life and Death

In a household, if you don't set simple, stable rules for living together, or don't respect them yourself, you're giving your child a very distressing living environment, subject to the arbitrary and volatile whims of each individual, the adult first. Children who seem all-powerful grow up to be anguished beings. Hans went through a real phobic illness. It's difficult and stressful to survive in the jungle.

Parents who come to me to ask their child to listen to them are always very surprised to find themselves forced to do some practical work where they have to learn to be consistent with their own injunctions. To announce only what they can keep, and keep what they announce.

It's much easier to say in September that there won't be any presents at Christmas - which makes no sense at all - than to refuse a toy every time you go to the supermarket!

And what about the illusory threat of boarding school for a five-year-old when his parents can't ask him to give up his third dessert?

Authority means knowing how to say "no" to yourself and respecting your own word.

Authority means being able to govern yourself.

The lack of authority that lets children drift as they please sometimes amuses parents during the first two years, as the child takes liberties. But the situation can quickly become unmanageable, ending in reciprocal violence between the child - who accepts no frustration - and the parent - who believes he or she has no educational leverage other than physical restraint - and the child.

10.
Angélique has Won her Freedom

But his parents didn't hit the jackpot

While the facts evoked are real, the documents reproduced and the places and names cited are fictitious. This is a transposition of this child's story.

Welcomed into the children's home, Angélique came regularly to the nursery to help care for the babies, on an apprenticeship, you might say. She was fourteen at the time. She was assiduous, a good listener, attentive and skilful. Here are a few elements of her story, arranged in an intelligible chronological order.

Article from the newspaper *La Libre Province*, May 24, 19**:

"Another road tragedy has plunged our department into mourning. A family of three children, living in B., was involved in a sad traffic accident yesterday morning. Their car was hit by a heavy goods vehicle in circumstances that the shocked driver was unable to explain. The S. fire department quickly arrived on the scene, only to discover that the mother of the family had died. The father and his three young children, more or less seriously injured, were evacuated to La V hospital. According to the latest information, their lives are not in danger. The editorial team extends its deepest condolences to the family and wishes a speedy recovery to the injured."

Eighteen months later :

Article from *La Libre Province*, Saturday, November 26:
"[...] a thirty-nine-year-old man was imprisoned on Friday at the Moulin-Carré prison in N. [...] Shortly after his wife's death, a thirteen-year-old niece, still a schoolgirl, came to help him with household chores and the upbringing of his three young children. It wasn't long before the teenager shared his adult life. Completely. An inspector from the Department of Health and Social Intervention alerted the public prosecutor in N.: the child was more than two months pregnant with her uncle's child. A confrontation is scheduled for Monday..."

A few days earlier :

October 31:
Report from the Director of the Social Intervention and Solidarity Department to the Public Prosecutor (extracts):
"The school social worker, alerted by repeated absences from school, observed that fourteen-year-old Angélique M. had been living intermittently with her maternal uncle

by marriage, with her parents' agreement, for nearly four months. Angélique M. is described as a rather withdrawn young girl. Her uncle, Mr. Julien C., admitted having had sexual relations with his niece, and that she was pregnant. He also stated that he would like to live with her. Angélique's parents accept this state of affairs and are completely unaware of their parental responsibilities.

Angélique was able to tell the social worker that she didn't like school and didn't want to live with her parents any more because of the constant arguments. Angélique explained that her uncle and his children needed her presence, and that she was happy to help them. She added that her uncle's three children loved her very much, and asked for her, and that Mr. Julien C. was tired of having to rely on domestic workers to look after the house and children. She also stated that other cousins had come to help Julien C. before her, that it was a family rule to help each other and that her uncle had always been very fair to all of them.

The school social worker met with the parents, who downplayed all the family difficulties alleged by Angélique, trivialized the school absenteeism and declared that the arguments only concerned the children between themselves...

An assistance measure for Angélique under child protection seems necessary..."

X. juvenile court, order of November 10:
"We, F. Timme, Juvenile Judge, acting pursuant to the provisions of Articles 375 et seq. of the Civil Code, and Articles 1181 et seq...

In view of the urgency; whereas it is clear from the documents in the case file that the situation of this young teenager, who is said to be a few weeks pregnant with the child of her maternal uncle, appears to be particularly worrying; whereas it is necessary for her to benefit rapidly from a protective judicial measure in order, in particular, to provide her with the educational supervision and support which she currently appears to lack within her family;

For these reasons :

Entrust Angélique M. to the Direction des interventions sociales et de solidarité du département de X. as of November 12. Let us state that the social benefits to which the minor is entitled will be paid to the Direction des interventions sociales et de solidarité du département de X., etc."

November 21:

Gendarmerie report at the end of Mr Julien C.'s police custody.

"11/21/19** at 3:30 p.m.

We, the undersigned chief brigadier O. F., judicial police officer resident in S., being at our unit's office in S., accurately report the statements made before us by Mr. Julien C. at 3:15pm.

Statement of facts:

Mr. Julien C. admits having had sexual relations with the fourteen-year-old Angélique M., and claims to be the father of the unborn child. He specifies that he did not seek to abuse the young girl, just as he had been very correct with the other two nieces who had been sent to help him look after his three young children. 'Just ask them.' But that Angelique M. 'wanted to have him and she did' and that now 'he wants to marry her off'. When I reminded him of his age and that a marriage could not be contracted with a girl under fifteen, Mr. Julien C. told me that he had the agreement of Miss Angélique M.'s parents and that they would ask the mayor for a dispensation..."

November 22. Minutes of educational observations at the children's home:

"Angélique was admitted to the children's home yesterday Friday following the order of the children's judge. Angélique explained to the educators that she didn't want to go back to school and that her plan was to live with 'Julien' and raise her children. To our astonishment, she remained steadfast in this position. She didn't mention her pregnancy. She added that she no longer wanted to live with her parents because it wasn't easy, without elaborating. She did say, however, that since she had been living with her maternal uncle, one of her father's cousins had taken the liberty of squatting in her parents' room, and that she didn't like this character.

She was especially sad to be separated from her friend. She had tears in her eyes when she talked about it. If she was calm, she was revolted by what was happening to them: 'We haven't done anything wrong, what are they looking for us for, we just want to get married.'

Her anxiety grew as the day wore on, and she insisted on phoning the gendarmerie in S on her own. That's how she learned that her uncle, Mr Julien C, was in prison. She broke down in tears and refused to be seen by us. Later, she would express terrible anguish at knowing he was in prison, worrying about his condition. 'Why did they put him in jail and why did they lock me up here?' she asked.

In an attempt to appease him, we told him we'd call the gendarmerie back today, which we did. We learned from the brigade that a confrontation would take place on Monday.

This reassured Angélique that she would see her friend again within two days, and that she would be able to explain to the examining magistrate what had really happened.

November 24. Minutes of educational observations at the children's home:

"Angélique came to the confrontation with the examining magistrate in a very determined manner, telling us that she was responsible for what had happened, that she claimed to have been at the origin of their love affair and that they intended to live together. The examining magistrate dismissed the original charge of statutory rape against Julien C. and ordered his immediate release. Julien is now free, and the only prohibition he must respect is not to lodge Angélique in his home.

We're organizing a family planning appointment for tomorrow."

November 25. Minutes of educational observations at the children's home:

"Consultation at family planning for Angélique, who meets Mr. Julien C. We let them discuss the possibility of a voluntary interruption of pregnancy with the doctor and the psychologist. We let them discuss with the doctor and psychologist the possibility of a voluntary interruption of pregnancy."

November 27. Minutes of educational observations at the children's home:

"Angelique told us that she and her boyfriend had decided not to return to the family planning clinic for the second scheduled appointment, as they were determined to keep the baby. Mr. Julien C. confirmed this decision to the director of the home by telephone, who in turn informed the children's judge."

November 28th. Handwritten letter from Angélique M. to M. le juge des enfants:
"Mr. Juvenile Judge
I'd like to meet with you urgently to find out the reason I'm in the children's home."

November 29. Minutes of educational observations at the children's home:
"When her parents came to visit, Angélique refused to meet them. She went out into the corridor to tell them she didn't want to see them or stay with them. However, she rushed to answer a phone call from her friend's sister. Angélique then called Mr. Julien C. and insists on asking us when the judge will finally allow them to meet for a visit at the home."

December 2nd. Mr. Director of the Department of Social Intervention and Solidarity to Mr. Juvenile Judge:
"Your Honor,
Angélique M. is currently being cared for at the children's home, where in-depth work has been carried out on the unborn child and the possibility of a voluntary interruption of pregnancy. Angélique M. and Mr. C. were seen at the family planning center; following the interview, Angélique persisted in her desire to keep the child.
Angélique wants to meet Mr. Julien C. and has asked you for an appointment in order to get an answer to this question. I would like to point out, as indicated in the

social report of the children's home, that Angélique is very attached to Mr. C. and that it seems unrealistic to refuse to meet him..."

December 3. Minutes of educational observations at the children's home:
"We caught Angélique crying after she had a telephone conversation with her friend. We managed to figure out that Angélique's parents tried to extort money from Julien C."

December 4. Minutes of educational observations at the children's home:
"This time, the parents seek to pressure Angélique into convincing Julien C. to some dark transaction. Angélique confides little, but we sense that she is looking for ways to free herself from their grip. Is she beginning to see her pregnancy and marriage plans as levers that can be used to this end? She tests our reactions with selected brief confidences, and gauges our possible alliance in this undertaking."

December 10. Report on the meeting with the school social worker at the children's home:
"Mrs. B., a social worker at the N. secondary school, monitored Angélique's situation because of her absenteeism from school, which began at the end of the school year and had been increasing since the start of the new school year in September. Strangely enough, the parents were not concerned, taking it for granted that their daughter would move in with her brother-in-law to look after the children. When reminded of their daughter's compulsory schooling, they replied that they might have to ask Mr. Julien C. to send her to the local secondary school.

Mrs. B. also informed us that Mr. Julien C. had received a million from the opposing party following the accidental death of his wife. This was obviously a very large sum for the family. Mr. Julien C. was apparently quite lavish with his close relations, but this was carefully hushed up by the family and only discovered incidentally. A curatorship was set up to protect the children's assets. It is almost certain that financial motives were behind the waltz of Mr. Julien C's nieces. After his wife's death, he dismissed the paid care-givers he had been offered. Did the extended family send their young daughters to look after the children in return for payment? The undoubtedly uncalculated romance between Angélique and Mr. Julien C. certainly changed the situation and altered the balance of power. When this relationship was discovered by Angélique's parents, it was most likely the subject of a financial transaction - threats and blackmail by the parents against Julien C.? Had they monetized their marriage agreement? - They implicitly acknowledged having received several 'loans' from Mr. Julien C.

They continue to complain about the reduction in social benefits - the children's judge having ordered that these should no longer be paid to the parents, but placed in a separate account in Angélique's name, which they had not imagined possible and which thwarted their calculations - and they have also tried to claim that 'young mother' allowances should be paid to them - 'we are the little girl's parents', they say.

Mrs. B. also reports her surprise at Angélique's complete turnaround when her pregnancy was discovered. When it was announced, whereas up until then she had been denying her relationship with her uncle by marriage against

10. Angélique has Won her Freedom

all the evidence, no doubt due to pressure from her family and the intervention of social services, she then showed herself to be extremely resolute, freeing herself from all these constraints, and asserting in a very determined way that she had no regrets, because it was her desire."

December 18. Minutes of educational observations at the children's home:

"Angélique comes to life when she talks to her educator about her relationship with Mr. Julien C. The sentimental dimension is clearly not the only thing Angélique discovers through this romance. She talks of her sense of freedom, her pleasure at being seen as responsible, and her gratitude for the affection shown to her by her friend's children. It's certainly a great contrast to the dull, difficult life she knew at her parents' home, which she still keeps quiet about, but which comes through during their visits.

During these meetings, to which Angélique sometimes resigns herself, she is passive and indifferent. The parents don't ask any questions about the problems at home, the truancy, the complaints of one of the sons who would like to go to a home, or about the fact that a cousin on the father's side had taken advantage of Angélique's absence to squat in her room, and that they were unable to get him to leave. On the other hand, they returned to the subject of finances and the reduction in family allowances since Angélique's court-ordered placement.

When he talks about Julien and Angélique, her father displays a heavy, gravelly sense of humor that earns him angry looks from his daughter. On several occasions, we had to ask him to tone down his comments."

December 28. Minutes of educational observations at the children's home:

"Angelique spends hours on the phone with her boyfriend, and we had to make a rule about when and for how long these calls could tie up the office's only phone line. She refused a visit from her parents for Christmas.

Angélique has now named her father's alcoholism, but she finds it much more difficult to talk about her mother's, which seems to her shameful and against the nature of being a mother. She is very disappointed by this weak, cowardly mother, incapable of protecting her and indifferent to her real and serious questions as a child. Angélique told us that one of the reasons she decided to stay with her uncle and refuse to return to her parents was that her father's cousin, the one who had been squatting in her room, had tried to abuse her when she was younger. This apparently hadn't shocked the parents, who still welcomed this individual while urging Angelique to return home. She didn't feel safe with her parents.

The domestic climate of supposedly simple disputes between the children - as his parents claimed - now appears to be marked by verbal and sometimes physical violence between them, fanned by foolishness and alcohol."

January 12. Minutes of educational observations at the children's home:

"Angélique's parents would have dangled their agreement to the marriage in front of her, but Angélique doesn't believe a word of it. 'They say that on an empty stomach and then when they're drunk they phone Julien and all they do is insult him. They don't treat him like that because he made me a child, but it's that he doesn't give them money.'

She explains that Julien C. intends to use his money to buy a house with meadows and woodland. He wants to keep animals.

She lives through the ultrasound scans, but hides her condition from the other children and at school, where she has returned for a while. Now that she has interrupted her schooling, Julien is helping her with her correspondence courses."

January 20 :
"The Children's Judge to the Director of the Department of Social Intervention and Solidarity:
Further to your report dated 17 current concerning Angélique M., I have the honour of informing you that Mr. Julien C. has applied to me for access to his niece.
After having obtained the opinion of Mr. M., examining magistrate in N., it seems possible to me to authorize Mr. Julien C. to meet the minor on the premises of the children's home..."

February 4. Minutes of educational observations at the children's home:
"The parents refuse to sign for the opening of a bank account in Angélique's name. The children's judge contacted substituted himself for them and gave his authorization."

February 12. Handwritten letter from Angélique M.:
"Mr. Prosecutor,
I am writing you this little note to tell you that I agree to take Mr Julien C. in Marriage. As I am a minor, my parents have given their consent. Dear Sirs, I am asking you for an Answer so that we can get married as soon as possible.
Yours sincerely"

February 15. Minutes of educational observations at the children's home:

"How did she manage to get her parents to agree to the marriage? Mystery."

February 20. Letter from Julien C.'s guardianship delegate to the public prosecutor:

"Mr. Public Prosecutor,

As curator of the interests of Mr. Julien C. and his children, you have kindly requested my opinion on the appropriateness of an age waiver that would allow a marriage between Mr. C. and the young niece he has taken in.

One of the reasons for placing Mr. C. under curatorship was his excessive prodigality towards his family, which could have jeopardized his financial interests and those of his children. Mr. C. had received a very large sum from insurance following the accidental death of his wife, which could have given rise to covetousness, all the more so as he appeared very suggestible, this weakness of character no doubt being excused by the distress of having found himself alone with three young children. I'm therefore concerned about the consequences of such a union, which would have the effect of emancipating a teenager who has given a glimpse of a determined nature, no doubt capable of corrupting her uncle's judgment. There is a very real danger that this young girl will come to confuse her own interests and those of her unborn child with those of Mr. C.'s children, whom I am duty-bound to protect.

On the other hand, my role as representative of a federation of family associations, in my capacity as curator, leads me, in the face of a situation that offends the law, that morality condemns and that shocks the common understanding, not to advise favoring the regularization of such a union. On the other hand, it is not for me to express an opinion on the risk that would be represented by the continuation of a concubinage between a mature man and such a young girl, as this state does not confer any rights on the latter with regard to the financial management of the household, and this situation falls more within the prerogatives of a judge than those of a curator [...]".

March 4th. Monsieur le procureur de la République to Miss Angélique M. :

"I hereby inform you of my refusal to grant you the age exemption you are requesting to marry Mr Julien C. The reasons for this refusal are as follows: I do not consider it advisable to encourage a union between a fourteen-year-old girl and a man twenty-five years her senior. In addition, Mr. Julien C., who is your uncle by marriage, is the father of three children aged six, four and two respectively, whose mother-in-law you would become if you married Mr. Julien C. Here again, in your interest and that of your cousins, the union you are planning does not seem desirable to me.

Yours sincerely"

March 8. Social report from the children's home to the children's judge:

"[...] Angélique seems very detached from her parents, expressing no demands on them. During their visits, when she accepts to see them, she shows little affection, even displaying a certain harshness. She now discusses their alcoholism and criticizes them for focusing most of their discussions on financial matters. She also refuses to go to their house at weekends. The parents are visibly overwhelmed by events, and it's all the more difficult for them to show any lucidity as they are often under the influence of alcohol, whether it's Madame on the telephone, on several occasions, or even both of them during visits to the home [...].

[...] time spent in the nursery was set aside so that Angélique could familiarize herself with babies and the gestures and care to be given to a newborn [...]".

March 12. Extracts from the expert psychiatrist's report to the examining magistrate concerning Angélique M.:

"The girl is in good physical health, with no history of pathology. She has a good appetite, sleeps well, complains of no subjective disorders and is apparently coping well with her pregnancy. Her main concern is to find her boyfriend, from whom she suffers separation.

Examination of her mental functions did not reveal any serious alterations. Angélique has no provocative or seductive attitude. She has no tendency towards affabulation. Her intellectual capacities are at the lower limits of normal without being deficient. She has a fragile personality, characterized by a strong emotional quest and a search for protection, which we can attribute to the emotional deficiencies she seems to have suffered at the hands of her parents. What's more, her parents are said to be intemperate and to have violent marital conflicts. However, Angélique's young age and immaturity may have prevented her from realizing the validity of her choice of love, and from fully appreciating her future responsibilities as a mother [...]".

March 14 :

"Before the civil registrar of the town of B., Angélique
M. and Julien C. 'have declared that they recognize for
their child or children, the child or children of whom
Angélique M. declares to be currently pregnant.'"

March 15 :

Mrs C. (Julien C.'s sister-in-law) to the juvenile court
judge (in clumsy handwriting):
"Sir,
I am sending you this letter to ask you, please sir, if we
could receive Miss Angelique M. in our home. We have
room to sleep so for Angelique we are the future sister-
in-law and brother-in-law. Could you do the impossible? If
you see a small problem, there's also Julien C's mother-in-
law's house. Could you do the impossible?"

March 20.

Angélique M. to Monsieur le juge des enfants (in clumsy
handwriting):
"Mr. Juvenile Judge,
I am writing you this letter because I would like you to
receive me as soon as possible, because I would like to
ask you that during Mr. Julien C.'s visits we can leave the
Home, and I would like to know when I am going to leave
the Home. And if you don't want Mr. Julien C. and I to leave
the Home, I'd like to ask you to go to his mother's or his
sister-in-law's for the weekend".

March 25.

Monsieur le juge des enfants to Monsieur le directeur de la Direction des interventions sociales et de solidarité du département de X.:

"I have the honour of requesting that you acknowledge that I have no objection, unless you advise otherwise, to the requested permission for Mr Julien C. to leave the children's home during his visits to Miss Angélique M., without Mr Julien C. being able to take Angélique to her home."

March 27. Minutes of educational observations at the children's home:

"I accompanied Angelique to her ultrasound this morning. Angelique looked absolutely radiant. She's kept the photo prints with her and keeps looking at them.

I've never seen her so relaxed since she was admitted to the home. She was so reserved at first, but now she's mischievous, laughing and mischievous. She's always calling out to me, always wanting to come and talk to me. She tells me about Julien and the children. Insignificant things, but which show how much they are in her thoughts. Again, she shows me - 'look, look', she says - victorious, serene and light, the ultrasound photos.

I have the impression that she brandishes these Polaroids as a safe-conduct to her freedom, the fruit of chance and then of her struggle, which has become increasingly asser- tive over time, to escape her violent, alcoholic parents, pimps and putasers - 'And what's more, it's my grandmo- ther who dares to call me a whore', Angélique whispered to me - who only cared about their daughter's future to feed her to a sleazy cousin or try to sell her to a millionaire. They never had any consideration for her schooling or her well-being in family life.

But what is the cost of this freedom for Angélique? The price of an amputation of her youth: the loss of the carefree spirit of adolescence, but did she ever know it? The torpedoing of her schooling and professional future, but did her family even give her the ambition? A planned move away from home for several months, but wasn't living with her parents a more painful form of alienation? She reminds us of certain animals who, finding themselves caught in the jaws of a trap, end up mutilating their own leg to regain their freedom and keep their life. A desperate act to survive.

Angélique leaves us tomorrow to go to the Foyer de N."

Epilogue

As a result, Angélique was exiled to a remote town and placed in a boarding school for pregnant teenagers, a modern version of the convents of yesteryear where young girls from good families who had erred were welcomed. The rules are strict, visits limited and outings forbidden. The monastic rules of yesteryear have been replaced by the modern laws of hygiene, psychology and education. Four months later, she gave birth to a little girl, Julie, whom "she looked after calmly and with great care", as the home's educators explained to the juvenile court. Her boyfriend comes to visit her every weekend with his children.

He was eventually convicted and imprisoned for a few weeks, as punishment for his relationship with Angélique. When he was released from prison, she obtained permission from the juvenile court judge to spend weekends at his home with her baby. It was during one of these trips that we were surprised to see Angélique and her little Julie again.

Taking advantage of the time between the train that had brought her from the city of her exile and the bus that would take her to her friend's house in the depths of the département, she had spontaneously come to the children's home to introduce us to her little girl, under the pretext of having forgotten her diapers. It was a moving and joyful encounter, full of laughter and cries, followed by silence so as not to wake the little girl. Afterwards, she picked up her child and her bundle and headed off to the bus station to board an omnibus coach to join her man.

Soon, this exile becomes too much, and Angélique runs away with her child from the home for young teenage mothers to stay with her boyfriend. On the eve of her fifteenth birthday, the juvenile court judge ratified the situation, granting Julie's father the right to take in her mother as well. They then went to the town hall to declare themselves cohabitants.

Angélique was still a minor, neither married nor emancipated, and the law being the law, thanks to the release of the children's judge, it was her parents who finally received the family allowance.

Despite the number of children who have been looked after by the child welfare services - over six hundred thousand in the under-18 age group, or perhaps a total of over two million adults - the public and the general public only know about the reality of these children's lives through news stories, as in the case of Angélique. These are sometimes extraordinarily dramatic stories that make the front pages of newspapers and the media, of which children are most often the victims (cases of paedophilia, infanticide or conflicts between parents, foster families and authorities) and, very rarely, the actors, through criminal acts; when the latter involve certain adults, it is never forgotten that they have passed through the "Dass". The mass of these children is far more suffering and silent than asocial and delinquent.

For most of them, child welfare services represent a refuge and a rescue, and often their only emotional ties. The task of improving their care remains immense and sometimes discouraging. But on the other hand, the progress made over the last century has been just as remarkable, in terms of the quality of the care they receive, their medical and educational follow-up, and in the quest for greater consideration for their families.

But these hundreds of thousands of children remain hidden under a bushel, and their fate is of little concern to many. Yet it's an inescapable reality that raises essential questions for our society. An American pediatrician, outraged by the general lack of concern for these neglected children, whether on the part of doctors, the school community or politicians, even wrote a vengeful article entitled *Neglecting the Neglect of Neglect*[38].

Ordinary parents with educational difficulties are also unaware that they can find help from Child Welfare professionals all over the country... without risking their child's placement!

---

38. Dubowitz (H.), "Neglecting the neglect of neglect", *Journal of Interpersonal Violence*, no. 9, 1994, pp. 556-560.

11.

LÉNA REFUSES TO EAT

Are you sure you're not raping your child?

Willy was two years old. His pediatrician, concerned about his retarded intellectual and language development, his incoercible tantrums and his stubborn character, had referred him to my consultation. His condition would not have been too alarming in an ordinary family who would have understood the need for psychological care and a coherent education, but Willy was being brought up by an intellectually deficient mother who did as she pleased, disregarding educational or medical advice which - depending on her good or bad will - she neither heard nor understood.

The most telling example was that of the "Chinese shoes". Unable to find her way around sizes, Willy's mother had bought him a pair of shoes she thought were magnificent, but which turned out to be too small. Despite this fatal flaw, she was adamant that her son should wear them, because she was very proud of her "Made in China" purchase. The result was that Willy walked with little steps, grimacing like a Chinese girl with bandaged feet, or refused to put them on at all, two behaviors that soon made us discover not only the incongruity - which brooked no discussion - between feet and shoes, but above all his mother's obtuse and obstinate character. She continued to impose these beautiful shoes on Willy, despite the repeated remarks of the pediatrician, the educator and myself, as well as the evidence of Willy's walking difficulties.

Other neglects in his upbringing and basic care only increased and became so alarming that the juvenile court judge decided to entrust Willy to a foster family.

Nevertheless, despite her obvious incompetence in many areas, this mother wisely acknowledged her inability to do anything about her son's temperamental behavior, and complained about it.

"He doesn't listen to me, he just does what he wants.

I asked her about it, and she explained her problem very naturally:

- Willy sleeps in a little bed next to mine. Now that he can walk well, he's able to get out of his and climb onto mine. Then he climbs on top of me and lies down on top of me, his belly on top of mine and he goes han! han! han! moving back and forth as if he wanted to make love to me. And he gets a hard-on - she laughs a little, half amused, half embarrassed. I don't want to. I tell him, "No, Willy! No Willy!" But he doesn't listen to me and goes on and on. As soon as I want to go to bed, he climbs on my bed and says "Bisou! Bisou!" I think he wants a kiss to go to sleep, but he starts climbing on me again. How do I get him to stop?

- But where did he learn this?

- Well, I don't know. Maybe he sees us do it when my boyfriend comes over. My boyfriend often comes in the afternoon during Willy's nap and that's when we make love. In the evening, he's at his wife's. Several times Willy has wanted to climb into bed with us and we've scolded him to stay in his. Since then, when my boyfriend is here - my boyfriend has a big voice - Willy doesn't flinch, he stays in his bed. I can see it: he pretends to be asleep. But as soon as I'm alone with him, he starts climbing all over me again. You'd better tell Willy not to do that to me. It's really embarrassing.

Here's a mother incapable of setting any limits for herself. She won't give up her little-girl whim of buying those shoes and admit how small they are. She refuses to set limits on her love affair and continues to make love in front of her son. Unable to govern herself, how could she possibly be able to sct an cducational framework for Willy in the ordinary situations of life? She sees herself as even more helpless in these unsavory circumstances. And yet, she seems to have a certain perception of the prohibition of incest.

Léna was placed in the nursery at the age of four months. The children's judge had ordered her placement and that of her three-year-old sister, due to a climate of educational confusion - the term is weak - and serious lack of care.

In Léna's case, it was her eyes that struck me first. Eyes so big they ate her face, an otherwise empty face, smooth and expressionless. In all circumstances, her intense vigilance was concentrated in those huge eyes. On the lookout.

Maëlle, her family assistant, had been very touched by this little girl who was so anxious, so fearful, who wouldn't let herself go in her arms, who couldn't bear for faces to come close to her, and who would only accept to be carried with her back against you, her sharp eyes scanning the surroundings. Feeding this sickly baby, who was only half her theoretical weight, was an ordeal. The little one never asked for food, so much so that she feared for her life at the slightest illness. She refused to let anything approach her lips or mouth. If her nurse tried to insert the bottle's nipple between her lips, however carefully, Léna would struggle. Hungry, she sometimes agreed to drink, but soon interrupted the feed and rejected the still half-full bottle. She advanced in age, grew a little, but her weight stagnated dangerously. Medical examinations gave no explanation for her refusal to feed.

When Léna was around eight months old, during her parents' weekly visits, her childminder observed some stupefying behavior on the part of the baby's mother. These parental meetings took place in a center under the supervision of a social worker. But the reunions or goodbyes were sometimes less controlled, under Maëlle's gaze alone. The mother, who had noticed these moments of vacation from the social services, exploited them. Taking advantage of these moments of hesitation, she prolonged the greetings, for her own benefit, while Léna sought instead to return to her nurse's arms. One day, the mother became a little bolder and, after turning to check that the social worker was out of sight, she pounced on her daughter in the arms of her childminder. She pounced on Léna like a forbidden fruit, saying "Bisou! Bisou!" Then she snogged Léna and stuck her tongue in her mouth. A real puke-inducing galosh for an eight-month-old baby! Surprised, her nanny retched and could only stammer out:

- But you can't do that!

To which her mother replied without embarrassment:
- But Léna loves it.
Contradicting these words, Léna screamed!
Maëlle's heart is still in the right place when she tells us about these events:
"She said Léna loved it, but Léna screamed! So, besides, given the aplomb of her answer, it was a habit for her. This wasn't a furtive little kiss on the lips as might be seen in some families, but a real scoop with the tongue. It was forceful, voracious, intrusive, violent. The mother took pleasure in it, an owner's pleasure that showed whose master she was. It was an act of affirmation of her enjoyment as owner. Physical possession as an act of ownership and territorial domination. A rape of war. This child was her thing and she was exercising her right to enjoy it. It shouldn't be called a kiss; the word *kiss* means tenderness, but I don't have another word for it. Although, hearing me say it like that, the word *kiss* could be taken as a verb. It wasn't a gesture that could be described by a common noun, but an act that required a verb to define it.

Kissing.

And to add to the confusion, the mother would say, 'Bisou! Kiss!'

My heart was beating a mile a minute."

Maëlle stops for a moment, looks at us, straightens up, sighs and continues:

"I'm almost ashamed to have to tell you all this, but I need to talk about it, I can't keep it inside me. I took Léna to her first appointment with her child psychiatrist. I introduced her to Léna and told her what I've just told you.

It was this doctor who, before me, used the word *rape* and I think she's right. She added that she thought this mother loved her child, but that she loved him with a horrible love.

I was reminded of other observations that had surprised me on previous visits. Before leaving, Léna's mother would always tuck her head under the hood of the baby carriage, which immediately made her daughter scream. She was certainly taking advantage of her hidden position to roll her daughter's skates. I was also amazed that, as she grew older, Léna, instead of holding out her arms to her mother, brandished them forward to push her away. This must have been why Léna had adopted the position of a lookout, with her back against me and her hands out in front. With her little arms, she defended herself as best she could from her mother, who did not hesitate to impose these violent gallops on her.

Her father would tell her to leave her alone: 'You can see she doesn't want to', but the mother would reply: 'I need my dose! For two weeks!' The father would intervene, because he could see how the mother was bullying his daughter, but he didn't seem shocked that she would roll over on him. If Léna hadn't shown any signs of it, he probably wouldn't have felt the need to intervene.

I'd also noticed how brusquely she put her fingers in her daughter's mouth, 'looking for teeth', as if she were trying to retrieve marbles from a sink drain. What's more, her hands were dirty.

Léna wasn't gaining an ounce. I took her to the hospital for a check-up. Her parents were invited to attend. In the waiting room, I wanted to remain very professional and tried to engage in a minimum of dialogue with Léna's parents. But the subject of their daughter's progress didn't interest them at all. The small positive events in Léna's daily life that I tried to tell them about fell flat. Instead, her mother started talking about herself, and complained of having a sore throat. In an attempt to make conversation, I asked her if she'd seen a doctor. She replied:

'Oh no! At the doctor's it's: lie down and take off your thong!'

She laughed, proud of her verbal jibe, as she looked at the other patients in the waiting room. But as they all pretended not to have heard, she got up from her chair and began contorting herself, wiggling her buttocks in front of everyone as if something were tickling her pants.

'My zipper's stuck!'

She looked at the other bewildered parents, who were beginning to try and distract their little children from the show that was about to unfold, by gluing them to the pages of their old books.

Léna's mother pretended to start pulling down her pants, revealing her thong. The father wanted to intervene:

- Pull up your pants!

To which she replied:

- Ha! Ha! You want me to take off my thong? Ha! Ha! And I've also got my braces stuck.

All the other parents had suddenly become more short-sighted than the others: they had plunged their noses into their books and were reading them with their foreheads glued to the pictures.

She was as shameless in public as she was during her visits with Léna. And she paid no attention to Léna, who had come there for an essential consultation about her alarmingly low weight."

Léna's mother, unlike Willy's, is not marked by the prohibition of incest.

When stories like these pile up, sometimes you just can't breathe. To breathe a little, there are several solutions. Ignore it, move on and look away. Quickly forget about it and want nothing to do with it. Feel sorry for those poor parents and pity those unfortunate children. Revolt... against whom, against what? Everyone's looking for a solution.

I, too, probably needed a breather. In a first version of this text sent to my editor, I had gone on to give a long theoretical development on the family transmission of the incest taboo, on the irreconcilable differences between the taboo and the law, on the highly debatable concepts of social determinism and the transgenerational reproduction of behavior... Theorizing, another refuge.

I received an immediate e-mail in return: "And what became of them?"

Golly! That's the question! That's always the question.

These children are part of your life, and when you meet colleagues who knew one of them, the conversation quickly turns to their future. Painful developments and beautiful stories too. Many of these children have only professionals as family. But politicians and social service managers want to ignore this, moving, transferring and restructuring their staff. Rationalizing costs. Children don't care about ratios. I've known young adults who were "former ASE staff" who chose to move to keep pace with the transfers of social workers, to stay in their geographical area.

That's how I'd heard from Willy after he'd been placed in foster care.

His childminder reported that he had arrived at her home without any personal belongings. The only object he had brought from his mother's was a calculator, which he never parted with. He threw himself indiscriminately into anyone's arms. He had a panic fear of water: baths, showers, shampoos. He'd probably been ruthlessly washed. He ate with his hands and didn't know how to use a spoon. He rocked back and forth in bed to fall asleep, like the children in the orphanages of Ceausescu's Romania.

His mother never understood the need for placement, and refused with her stubborn little-girl stubbornness to come to the organized visits. He saw her only once again, fourteen years later.

Nevertheless, he went on to make good progress with his host family.

I had learned that he had started secondary school at the age of eleven and that his progress seemed satisfactory.

But that's without taking into account the upheavals of adolescence, when the rigged cards of early childhood are sometimes replayed.

The latest news I've received is much darker.

At the age of fifteen, Willy was given a suspended prison sentence and ordered to pay heavy damages for repeated sexual assaults involving threats and violence against a nine-year-old girl. He then had to leave his foster family. This was followed by a troubled period of repeated runaways from the home to which he had been admitted.

His mother died just before he came of age.

Then came signs of depression, numerous bodily anxieties and curious, offbeat comments. He tried to find out who his father was, without success. The family ties on his mother's side proved decaying.

After an episode of delirium, he was admitted to a psychiatric hospital. Due to an uncontrollable state of agitation, he had to be placed in an isolation room.

His psychiatrist suggests incipient schizophrenic psychosis.

This deterioration in his condition is undoubtedly not linked solely to the events recounted here. His criminal conviction at the age of fifteen and his exile from his foster family, the de facto abandonment of his mother and her untimely death, the absence of family ties on his mother's side and finally his fruitless research into his paternal filiation, all took their toll on his fragile psyche. A tragic destiny.

Could a parental lapse, made possible by de facto maternal abandonment when he was very young, followed by adoption, have changed the situation? Who knows?

And Léna?

Léna is now just over two years old. Maëlle gave me some fresh news:

"Good evening,

In response to your e-mail, here's some information.

Today, I'd say Léna trusts adults she knows well. Léna remains wary of strangers and comes to take refuge next to me. Only diapering remains difficult, at times: she stiffens up, squeezes her little legs and wiggles a lot. On the other hand, something new for some time now is that she cuddles me (and my husband) a lot, and takes our hands to stroke her hair.

She now eats a lot more, but on her own. Nevertheless, she no longer hesitates to ask the adults for help to finish a yoghurt, for example. She asks for food. When she sees grapes in the fruit bowl, she'll make herself understood and ask for them, even outside mealtimes. She's always selective, and often asks to eat what's on her neighbor's plate.

For the past three months, I've felt Léna much more tense around her parents' visits.

Before the visit: she's demanding, demanding my presence and my arms. Her tension is perceptible by all, since during a ride in the car, as I was re-explaining how

"Grown Ups are Really Stupid"

the afternoon was going to unfold, Bernard, a little three-year-old boy who is also in my care, exclaimed, 'But Léna doesn't want to see her mommy and daddy!' Léna refuses to walk to the social service premises. I have to carry her.

In the hall, I tell her again that we've come to see her mom and dad, and she always answers 'no! no!'

In the small room, separation is always difficult. Léna cries and refuses to go to her mom. However, she agrees to go to her father.

At the end of the visit, Mrs F. systematically wants to kiss Léna goodbye. Léna says 'no! no!' The mother takes no notice and kisses her anyway. But that's as far as it goes.

When we get back to the car, I keep Léna in my arms. She snuggles up to me and lets go completely. I can feel her soft little body.

After the visits, she found it difficult to fall asleep, staying up until nearly midnight on some evenings. On one occasion, she made herself vomit twice. What's glaring is that when she returns from the visits, she won't let go of me for the whole evening. I have to hold her in my arms until she goes to bed.

In terms of language, she's starting to say words: she said 'Daddy' when showing her father's photo.

At the moment, I think she's progressing at great speed, I find her cheerful, bubbly, with a thirst to grow! [...]"

Léna was placed in care much younger than Willy and learned to say "no". She was able to protect herself and rely on reliable guardians early on. I can only hope that her future will be less bleak.

12.

Martin is Either his Father or a Stone

If you're too intrusive, you'll swallow your child.

"A beautiful baby weighing one hundred and twenty kilos, but unpredictable and impressive when he gets angry." That's how the child welfare worker describes this "difficult" father.

A difficult father! The professionals soon found out. The judge was insulted and intimidated with his fist on the desk during the hearing, but did not react. The head of department was jostled, mobbed and blown into the bronchi as he left the courtroom. Fortunately, he was not alone, which prevented a more serious gesture. And an educator was threatened with physical reprisals against her children. "And you, I know where you live, was it your daughter I saw? The house with the green door is your home, you'll see, I'm going to sting you," he threw in her face, mimicking a knife wound.

Her son, Martin, has just been placed in care at the age of three. He is virtually speechless, expressing himself only through noises or isolated words. He relieves himself in his pants, and is fearful and frightened. His five-year-old sister was placed with him at the same time. She's a very anxious child, mute, with a serious, closed face, who fears adults and shows a delay in all her acquisitions and development. Her hair is very long, dirty, untangled and covered in lice. Her nails are broken and black.

When you address him, Martin freezes. For no discernible reason. Stunned, he looks like a complete idiot. His eyes stare at you without seeming to understand anything. Petrified, he doesn't answer your questions, not even with a nod. But his eyes stare back at you. Eyes wide open, but empty: you can see right through them, and they absorb you. You don't know whether he's imploring, questioning, worried, stupid, brainless, dumbstruck or maybe just lost. If you insist too much, his eyes roll back and his gaze turns white. Blind? Deaf? Dumb? Stupid?

Martin's father has obtained permission from the judge to take him home at weekends. When he returns from these outings, Martin sometimes speaks, but hidden, huddled, invisible, behind a sofa. One day, an educator even worried that she'd lost track of him. He didn't answer her calls, until she discovered him prostrate.

From his hiding place, Martin could have said, "A peur.[39]" But we don't know what of.

Sometimes, when he returns, his father is very proud to recount the weekend's activities:

- The other week, I took him to the garden center. There were Santa's decorations. Santa was snoring in a wooden shack. You could see him breathing and snoring. The red

---

39. Scared.

coat on his big belly, going up and down. Martin, that gave him the willies! It made me laugh! How can anyone be afraid of Santa Claus? Martin wanted to run away. I told him to stay there and watch!

What I said to Martin: Santa Claus, you see, he's snoring, but he won't always be sleeping. When he wakes up, he'll come home. And you know what he's gonna bring you. He'll bring you diapers for Christmas, if you're not clean and still shitting your pants.

The Martin had scared the shit out of him. So this week, I went to see him again. That way, he wouldn't feel like shitting his pants.

I don't give a damn about him when he pisses his pants, I just laugh and tell him: you stink! you stink!

The educator tried to interrupt:

- Ah! That's probably why he's been having nightmares all week. He told us he was afraid of "Christmas". We didn't know what it was. Maybe you should...

It probably wasn't the kind of remark to make to her. He stepped forward, suddenly menacing. Under the circumstances, his stature and stoutness were quite impressive. He raised his chin and his tone, white with rage:

- You're not going to explain to me what I should or shouldn't do. Because first of all, even the judge only does what I say. At the home, all of you didn't want Martin to come for the weekend. I never hit Martin! The judge didn't listen to you. He listened to me! I'm the father!

Martin, who had witnessed the scene, had discreetly taken cover behind the educator. The father suddenly turned around and disappeared without a word, without a goodbye.

Martin's pants were all wet.

12. Martin is Either his Father or a Stone

During the week, Martin stays with his childminder, Sophie. At her place, Martin relaxes a little and begins to enjoy being with her. He always stays close to her, but doesn't ask for affection. To protect Martin from the anxiety of seeing her worried by this father, weekend departures and returns are organized at the home. A safety lock.

One Saturday, Martin's father is waiting for him in a small room. He reads the newspaper. The educator arrives with Martin. The father doesn't look up from his reading. Martin freezes and doesn't know what to do. So the educator tries to start a conversation. Martin doesn't know what to do, so he stays back. The father says nothing. He gets up, walks over to Martin, but doesn't hug him: he shakes his hand, without a word.

They're leaving.

The next day, the father is furious:

"Martin y'a me parlé de la grosse vache. What do they call her? Sophie? Is that it? And Sophie here and Sophie there! I don't want him to tell me about Sophie!"

He approaches the educator and glares at her.

Another educator, alerted by the escalating tone, makes himself visible to prevent a physical escalation. Martin runs to take refuge behind the educator, which only serves to redouble the father's anger.

"If this keeps up, I'll be back with my forty cousins to beat the shit out of all of you!"

Suddenly, he lowered his gaze and spoke in an imperative tone to Martin, desperate and sheltered. He hadn't even said hello to him the day before:

"Say goodbye to Daddy!"

Martin, frozen, staring at him with his big, inexpressive eyes.

"Martin, you're going to say goodbye to Dad!" he starts shouting.

Martin doesn't move an eyelash, no sound leaves his lips, he's emptied from the inside.

"If you don't come and say goodbye, I'll kill your goldfish!"

And he leaves, just as abruptly.

This time, Martin pooped his pants.

Martin is getting used to life with Sophie. But he's a child who's complicated to understand and always changing. Sophie never knows which character she's going to be dealing with.

Martin is not a very "demonstrative" child. He hasn't known hugs or kisses and doesn't ask for them. Just a little sometimes in the evening and when he's separated.

Martin's speech is improving, his vocabulary is expanding and his sentences are better constructed, but he's still difficult to understand. He hides behind the sofa and acts out skits. He alternates between different voices, which is surprising given his language delay.

In a thick, hoarse voice that comes from the back of his throat, guttural and nasty:

"Don't make a mess! Daddy's sleeping! Daddy, his leg hurts! Don't make a mess! I can't hear the TV."

In a higher, whispered, but imperative voice - no doubt her mother:

"Daddy's going to bed! Be quiet! Don't wake Daddy!"

Then, in a deep, guttural voice once again, Martin scolds and berates his doudou, who is flying over the sofa.

If the TV's on, he suddenly starts whispering.

All these characters invade the space of his thoughts and games, even from a distance. They have taken possession of his inner world.

12. Martin is Either his Father or a Stone

Little by little, Martin allows himself more freedom with Sophie. When he returns from weekends, he can now talk about certain things. Mostly, he talks about the things that scared him.

But often, Martin still freezes as soon as she addresses him, for a small instruction or a light reprimand. No way to get anything out of her. A real stone. Sometimes, it's no longer fear he feels, but a look of hatred.

For no reason at all, Martin can insult Sophie copiously in incomprehensible galimatias. He looks aggressive, makes a fist, puffs out his chest, runs around the house, rolls his eyes like a madman, contracts in on himself, clenches his fists. Sophie, with her calm, serene temperament, doesn't take these rantings seriously, nor do they seem directed at her. She's almost amused by them without showing it; if Martin now dares to play the big man, it's because he feels safe with her. This is not a house where things suck!

But misfortune! Martin must have allowed himself to use this galimatias at his father's house. He's not even aware that this ersatz insult was inspired by his own tirades.

Back from the weekend, the father is in a rage. But for once, he calls the educator to witness. He seeks her support: progress at last?

"Martin says bad words there. Did he learn that at Sophie's? I told Martin that if he keeps on swearing, we'll cut off his willy."

Martin looks at him with his big, coy eyes.

The following Tuesday is the day of the routine medical check-up with Colline, the department's pediatrician. Sophie had informed him the day before. Martin knows Colline well; she's very gentle and patient with the children.

In the morning, Sophie gets Martin ready. But he becomes irritated, then hostile.

He shouts. He doesn't want to go:

"I'm not sick."

Sophie manages to dress him. Martin runs away. He takes off all his clothes. He runs to hide. Tension mounts.

Sophie explains that it's time, that she has no choice and neither does he. They're going to be late, they've had enough of capriciousness! That's enough! This is serious business. Besides, it's her job.

"Martin! Come here!"

Sophie tries to negotiate:

- You're going to play with Colline's tools, the stethoscope, the reflex hammer, the tongue depressors. Nothing doing. Sophie gets firmer. If you keep this up, there won't be any trouble tonight. No more results.

And, right away, Martin, who had stood behind the sofa in full view, said to him:

- I don't want to go to the doctor, he'll cut off my willy!

- What are you talking about? Where did you get this?

- Daddy told me that. That they were going to cut off my willy. Because of my pee-pee.

Real progress! Martin begins to confront the consistency of his father's threats with reality. Finally, he expresses his anxieties.

This doesn't stop Martin from continuing to "treat" Sophie.

It's often the day after a weekend at her father's that she observes him like this. In fact, when he behaves this way, he looks like his father," Sophie tells us.

Martin has a big stuffed toy, a big eeyore with big ears. He gets on his donkey, grabs its ears and goes "vroom! vroom!"

like his father on his scooter. Martin isn't just afraid of his father, he's fascinated by him too.

Martin is either his father or a stone. But he doesn't exist. Martin, whose surface oscillates between muteness and invective, does have an interior, which sometimes flows outwards. When his sphincters give out, that's when he's himself. It's his only authenticity. In silence.

Martin is three characters at once, taking turns on the stage of his days and fighting over his territory.

Martin-his father, whom he identifies with through violence and insults. It's then that the hatred in his eyes reappears.

Martin-la-pierre, when he's terrified, but sometimes also when he feels like opposing, which isn't such a bad sign.

Martin-le-petit, when he becomes a child again, confesses his fears to Sophie. But also when he calmly plays children's games.

Faced with the spectacle of his father's anger, Martin is inhabited by all three characters at the same time. The two sides of the same coin, and its thickness.

The obverse is Martin's father, the child fascinated and exalted by his father's omnipotence. This one is standing. His eyes are wide open, as if hypnotized.

The other side is Martin-la-pierre, the child terrified of being the object of this anger. His mouth is closed and his body frozen. His gaze unblinking.

Between these two, Martin-le-petit is the one who hides behind the educator. Slipped between the anger that fascinates him and the fear that petrifies him, there's little thickness available to him. Only his intestines and bladder prove that this little Martin still exists.

This splitting of the personality, this dissociation of the subject, is very dangerous, because the child cancels out his own nascent feelings and replaces them with those of the adult. It's a question of psychic survival. Not collapsing. In Martin's case, the internal emotion - *I'm afraid* - is replaced by exaltation - *I'm all-powerful* - an exogenous feeling. An irreconcilable internal contradiction. A trampling of the child's fragile thoughts by the adult's tyrannical shoes.

The effects of emotional abuse on children are easy to imagine. Loss of self-esteem, anxiety, inhibition, sadness, even depression. If denigration, suspicion, harassment and derogatory remarks can destroy an adult, *a fortiori* it's even easier with a child. Children trust adults. They don't have the means to question the words of someone who is their authority.

What is less well known is the great vulnerability of babies and young children to psychological abuse[40] - as in Martin's case - but also to situations of emotional chaos, de facto abandonment or the spectacle of domestic violence. These are situations of unpredictable and sometimes intertwined outbursts, deficiencies and uncertainties.

At birth, the human infant is totally dependent not only physically, but also psychologically on its mother or her

----

40. Although jurisprudence is beginning to use this term to describe certain acts of abuse, France still has no legal expression for psychological abuse, and it is necessary to refer to Quebec's Youth Protection Act to find a clear definition of psychological abuse: "When a child is subjected, in a serious or continuous manner, to behavior of a nature to cause him harm by his parents or another person, and his parents do not take the necessary steps to put an end to the situation. These behaviors include indifference, denigration, emotional rejection, isolation, threats, exploitation, including if the child is forced to do work disproportionate to his or her abilities, or exposure to domestic or family violence."

substitutes. They are very premature, both physically and psychologically, compared with other species. The baby is then unable to distinguish in the flow of emotions running through him - a baby is an emotional factory - what belongs to him and what belongs to the other, and which circulates between them in a kind of virtual umbilical cord carrying very real information[41]. It's a common belief that babies don't think. This is absolutely true. Babies use the adult's brain to think for them. But without knowing that the brain that responds to his messages is not his own, nor that the breast that feeds him does not belong to him. He will therefore internalize the adult's feelings and emotions, which can enlighten or trample on his own baby emotions.

It's only little by little that children discover the differences between themselves and others, through the little deviations and variations in their parents' responses to their needs. If his parents were too perfect, he would never discover their otherness! It's the appearance of the "no" that signals this second birth and the detachment of the psychic placenta, which "releases the mother" as Winnicott writes. This expulsion[42] is not always a deliverance for the parents! In fact, it marks the beginning of the tantrum and opposi-

---

41. In this virtual umbilical cord between mother and child and between child and mother, psychic information circulates through the various channels of voice and speech, exchanged glances, carrying and skin contact, also known as "early interactions". The fluidity of emotions, the warmth of separations and reunions, and the regular pulsation of the little rhythms of daily life also gradually build up a prosody of the relationship. The expression "he or she hasn't cut the cord" is a metaphorical trace of this state.

42. In obstetrics, the expulsion of the placenta a few minutes after childbirth is called "delivery".

tion period, when the child experiences and exploits with glee the understanding of his difference from the other, and practices self-assertion.

This is why the human baby is so vulnerable during the very first months of life. He or she feels very strongly the emotions, feelings and thoughts of adults, but does not yet know how to distinguish between what is his or her own and what is not[43].

He has no way of defending himself against it, or protecting himself if necessary. He has no way of thinking "no", let alone saying it.

If the adult's intentions, words or actions are inappropriate, toxic or malevolent, they contradict the child's needs and emotions. With its physical survival at stake due to its dependence on others, the child will cancel out its emotions and thoughts to remain in symbiosis and survive. He will then appropriate the adult's emotions by denying his own. For the child, the only possible way to overcome the ordeal is to adopt the aggressor's emotions so as not to be destroyed. To survive, they must give up all thought of their own.

---

43. This experience of psychic confusion, known as "primordial transitivism", can be found in the dream of being able to read minds, in the memory of fleeting experiences of thought transmission, in the feeling of psychic fusion in the passion of love, or even in the popular communion of sports, music or art crowds. These few examples of shared identity are far from exhaustive.Shortly after psychic release, the child may remain "clinging", with difficulty in assuming psychic autonomy, also known as "individuation". It is at this stage of development that we observe periods of iterative questions addressed to the adult every few minutes, as if the child were seeking to regain a lost psychic closeness. This is the period of "why?" and "what's that?" or "are you okay?" repeated a hundred times during the day.

It's this gap between the reality of his needs and the nature of his thinking - which is not yet his own, but which is taking shape - that will be very destructive.

It's a kind of Stockholm syndrome - described in 1978 by the American psychiatrist F. Ochberg - of the child towards its parent. In fact, the description of Stockholm syndrome, which concerns adults taken hostage, proves that in vital situations, mature people can regress to this level of archaic functioning. The hostage cancels out his or her own thinking and adopts that of the captor - the ambiguity of the term becomes clear - in the hope of escaping. In fact, it's a common technique for hostage-takers to use their prey as messengers of their demands. The prey becomes the aggressor's spokesperson. We also encounter this phenomenon with children confronted by parents who are followers of a sect and who ritualize their relationship with the child according to their ideology, without taking into account the child's thoughts or needs. A real brainwashing.

When an adult is destabilized by psychological abuse, he or she may become aware of it, criticize it and complain about it.

The child experiences this as justified severity, since, in principle, adults are there to protect and guide him.

But the younger the child, the more serious the consequences, as it affects the very construction of their psyche.

I've known children who attacked their bodies as a result of clearly identified psychological abuse perpetrated by their parents. I remember Brice, who at the age of four defenestrated himself from the second floor after his violent father ordered him to run away from the children's home. Gaël, who seriously injured himself during a state of agitation in reaction to his mother's delirium, which announced fanciful and changing filiations.

"A fortnight ago, I told you that your father was Peter. But then I met Paul, and seeing his hands and feet that look like yours, I think he's your father."

And Claude, who at the age of six had become the scapegoat of his schoolmates, mirroring what he was experiencing at home with his stepfather.

One might have seen them as the suicidal equivalent of escaping an overdose of stress. But this was not the case. In each case, it was a visible implementation on the body of the psychological abuse that was not visible. These children had internalized the violence inflicted on them, becoming perpetrators, actors and victims. They were self-destructing. This is even more dramatic.

Worse still, with very young children who internalize the family violence they are bottle-fed, and that which is practiced around them and on them, to the point of becoming very violent themselves in a hard-to-cure mimetic identification, which Maurice Berger[44] calls extreme pathological violence. We have received several of these children in our nursery. They require constant supervision.

Two years have passed.

As far as Martin's father is concerned, the situation has not changed much. He continues to try, with varying degrees of success, to manipulate the judge, the child

------

44. National Assembly, July 7, 2009. Minutes of March 17, 2009, pp. 133-146, *Rapport d'information fait au nom de la mission d'évaluation de la politique de prévention et de lutte contre les violences faites aux femmes*, tome II, available at www.assemblee-nationale.fr/13/pdf/rap-info/i1799-t2.pdf

welfare officer and his son's and daughter's foster families. He manages to obtain abracadabra rights, but derisory in themselves, that no other parent would ever succeed in obtaining. Martin's mother is neither protective nor helpful. Intellectually limited, she is subservient to this man.

The three Martins are always at war. In their games, cars crash, houses burn and animals fight:

"They're bad guys."

His toys have a limited lifespan, and are quickly broken, dismantled and destroyed. He often tries to make trouble for Sophie, braves her, insults her again, opposes her and says "no".

But this Martin sometimes takes a vacation, more and more often, and now makes room for a curious, talkative little boy who asks questions all the time. During the former's absences, the other Martin sleeps well, no longer insults Sophie or seeks provocation. His cars are calmer, the dinosaurs are herbivores again and the men live in houses that don't burn down.

Although his language is still difficult to understand, his vocabulary is growing day by day. Martin is potty-trained at school and at Sophie's house, but the most frightening situations still end with a change of pants on the way home from his father's or on the first day at the day-care center.

Martin has begun to stand up to his father. The long practical sessions at Sophie's house, where he used to oppose her "for flan", are now bearing fruit.

Martin's paternal grandfather gave him a piece of clothing as a gift. His father and mother wanted Martin to give it to him. They categorically refused. Very upset, they ended up passing the new sweater on to Sophie, asking her to let him try it on "when he had made up his mind". The father was taken aback!

When Martin returned from his visits, he began to express himself. He understands that the proximity of other adults is a protection. He takes advantage of Sophie's presence to talk about what happened over the weekend. He still doesn't dare talk openly about himself, so he uses the subterfuge of staging his sister, whose fate is no more enviable. So, in front of his father, he managed to tell Sophie "Lina, she cried". No one was fooled; he was also talking about himself. The father, forbidden by such free speech that called him into question, could only respond with a double admission - "You don't have to say that, you snitch!" -a double admission of his responsibility and his inability to impose silence.

But that didn't silence Martin.

He continues to recount his little press review of visits to his father's house, each time he returns, in front of witnesses.

13.
STÉPHANE TOOK HIS FATHER'S CAR

Conditions for possible resilience

Stéphane enters and sits down. He's a composed, diligent young man whose permanent smile both masks and betrays his constant anxiety to be appreciated and recognized. He has come to see me following a *burn-out* syndrome that has literally destroyed him both psychologically and physically. He complains of heart palpitations and drops in blood pressure. He has lost several kilos and feels tired and listless. He finds it difficult to eat, and cannot contemplate returning to work.

Stéphane loved sales. As soon as he passed his professional exam, he immediately found a job. Looking to progress, he had moved on, changing employer and finally working in the fresh produce department of a supermarket belonging to a major distribution group, which, with a permanent contract in his pocket, should give him peace of mind. He had just passed his driving test and found himself a nice apartment in an old renovated farmhouse. He had even invited his colleagues from his previous job to come to the house-warming party, which, apart from the pleasure of receiving them, represented for him, in the spring of his twentieth year, the manifestation of his success and a nice revenge on life.

Then came the summer vacations. He found himself alone in charge of his department, trouble piled up and a colleague took a dislike to him. Exhaustion was already threatening, but he hung in there. It was then that a notary contacted Stéphane to inform him of his father's death and to ask him for certain information needed to settle the estate. After work, he had to go and sort through the house his parents had hated. The pressure, fatigue and memories overwhelmed him. He fell unconscious twice at work and ended up in hospital.

It was when he was released from hospital that he came to see me, or should I say, came *back to* see me. In fact, I had known Stéphane since he was a child, as I happened to be the child psychiatrist at several of the institutions that had taken him in.

Today, dejected and on sick leave, he declares himself very disappointed not to have held his place to the end in the job he had wanted and obtained, where he had been appreciated for his efficiency and seriousness. "It's sad not to be like the others. I'm too tired and it's no fun. But I did everything I could. I thought I was going to make it and now I'm devaluing myself and feeling ashamed. And that, added to all the difficulties of my childhood, is impossible to accept. I've recovered from the delays of my early childhood and my difficulties at school, but not from this fragility… I would have liked my work to finally bring me the pride and recognition to forget this childhood of hardship."

As he talks about the difficulties of his young adult life, memories come flooding back. Stéphane had been taken into the nursery of the children's home at the age of four months, taken away from his mentally ill mother, who was unable to look after him. It was his fifteen-year-old older sister who provided the bare minimum of care for this fragile baby. Indeed, within minutes of his birth, Stéphane stopped breathing due to a sudden withdrawal from the enormous doses of hypnotics, neuroleptics, sedatives and antidepressants his mother had been taking, combined with massive tobacco intoxication. Stéphane, totally drugged by all the products he had been immersed in for nine months, couldn't breathe. He remained hooked up to a machine for two weeks, and then spent a further two months in hospital. His development was reassuring at the time, and there was nothing in his physical or mental state to prevent his discharge. His mother came to see him very little during his hospitalization, apparently overwhelmed by the problems of adapting to everyday life. Getting on the bus to return to the hospital five stations later seemed an insurmountable adventure. However, despite the medical team's hesitations, Stéphane was handed over to her after hospitalization, in exchange for a promise that she would be supported by a home carer offered by the social services. Stéphane was two months old at the time.

A few weeks later, the attending physician, worried that he hadn't seen the baby in consultation since his return home, went to see his mother, but was loudly rebuffed. The social worker who had suggested home help received the same response. Stéphane's mother, in a state of patholo-gical psychic exaltation, refusing all care for herself and not caring for her children for several weeks, was then hospitalized in a psychiatric ward. Stéphane and his older sister were then placed in a children's home.

On his arrival at the nursery, four-month-old Stéphane was very passive and unresponsive. He seemed sad and uninterested in his environment. He only showed signs of hunger with very uncoordinated movements, but lacked energy and an appetite for life. He never cried. He never handled any objects, and spent much of his time sleeping. He didn't respond to the caregivers' requests and showed no emotion, neither pleasure nor displeasure. When picked up, he was very limp, did not hold his head like other babies of his age, and slid between the hands like a sound doll. Only his eyes were still present. It was a gaze that scrutinized, observed, but remained inexpressive. Stéphane was attentive to everything going on around him, but nothing seemed to disturb or animate him. It was a gaze that did nothing but watch. If an adult's gaze became too insistent, his would slowly drift away to avoid it. It seemed to freeze and retract in on itself when someone moved towards it, without taking infinite precautions to warn and reassure it. Worry, even fear, would be the first emotions he would express. It was a behavior akin to infantile autism, but in this case, it was a kind of experimental autism provoked by a great affective and sensory deprivation during the two months he spent with his mother. It wasn't until he was ten months old that real smiles and a few chirps appeared. At fifteen months, he was unable to stand up and could only crawl, leaving his legs dragging behind him. At this sight, the nursery's new nurse, who had come from a rehabilitation center for the handicapped, thought he was paraplegic. He walked much later.

Only his sister came to see him regularly. The mother occasionally visited him, but showed no emotion or affection, asked for no news or information about his development, and remained very distant from the baby, who didn't seem to interest her.

A few months later, Stéphane was taken in by a foster family, where he remained beyond the age of majority. However, this placement was called into question several times during his childhood, according to the vicissitudes of changing social workers and juvenile court judges, professions subject to the influences of cyclical variations in educational and psychological theories on the necessity or otherwise of maintaining a link, and in what form, with the natural parents.

Stéphane remained a very insecure little boy, always cautious in front of others, with a significant delay in all his acquisitions and development. He didn't start talking until he was three. He would remain withdrawn in the face of new situations, very quickly becoming anxious and developing very strong phobias, for loud noises in particular. He had an uncontrollable fear of dogs, and the sight of one, even when locked up, could leave him petrified, absorbing all his energy. He would become elusive, cutting himself off from reality and the person he was with.

Psychological care was quickly put in place at the nursery - this is when I met him - and continued until his adolescence. His psychomotor retardation and a certain slowness in communication would take years to diminish, without disappearing altogether. This would prove to be a serious handicap in his studies and professional life, where he would have to make extraordinary efforts to achieve sufficient efficiency. But Stéphane wanted to have a life like everyone else, and showed surprising energy to overcome his difficulties, which he paid for by losing his job through exhaustion. The constant, discreet but effective support of his foster parents was a solid support and a real opportunity for him. He will always be grateful to them.

One particular episode, from which I learned a lot, is still very vivid in my memory.

Stéphane was six or seven at the time. This was in the nineties, when the dominant ideology of the day was that of maintaining ties at all costs between children in care and their parents. The child welfare social worker seemed to be an active proponent of this "return home" theory. With his support, the parents were able to have the child at home at weekends. The social worker felt that this was a preliminary stage to his return to his family, which he considered possible and desirable: his parents had been cooperative, and the information gathered about how the weekends went seemed reassuring. His psychological care continued, and he was brought every week by his foster family for consultation at the psychological care center where I worked. Stéphane remained a self-effacing, shy little boy, with few opportunities for self-expression.

With my team, we wondered whether the parents would be able to adhere to this therapy and ensure the continuity of this essential psychological care themselves if the judge decided to return Stéphane to them. We therefore invited them to an appointment in the department to assess this question.

On the day in question, Stéphane arrived at the clinic ahead of them, brought by his family assistant. When he saw his parents, with whom he now regularly visited on weekends, enter the room, he didn't move towards them despite their invitation. He placed himself slightly to the side and behind the psychomotricist who usually received him for sessions. Half-hidden by his therapist's body, he gave her his hand discreetly behind his back. His little hand in hers. No one noticed. In the meantime, his parents were making promises that he would soon go home as soon as the judge decided. Looking at us in turn to make sure we were paying attention to the answer they expected from Stéphane, they asked him if he still agreed to come and live with them. This led us to assume that Stéphane had already been extensively briefed on this prepared speech, as the string was so thick. Stéphane shyly nodded his head in what appeared to be a "yes". But this little hand slipped stealthily and surreptitiously to a professional rather than to his parents had then enlightened us on Stéphane's deep insecurity towards them and on the fact that he didn't recognize them as guardian adults.

After their departure, Stéphane managed to explain to us that, in reality, he was very afraid of going to their home every weekend, and even more afraid of living there, but that he didn't dare say so in front of them. On the strength of these observations, we wrote to the juvenile court judge to express our concern that Stéphane should have to return under these conditions to parents he didn't recognize as such. Based on our opinion, the judge decided not to follow the proposals of the Children's Social Welfare Office and to keep Stéphane in his foster family.

Her parents, thus dismissed, abandoned their facade of unity, and reality set in. Madame, freed by the children's judge's decision, explained that her violent, alcoholic husband had terrorized her for a long time, but that she didn't dare complain for fear Stéphane wouldn't be returned to them. With this admission, she left the marital home for a few months. For his part, Stéphane explained the terror he felt at his father's violence, and the fear he felt at his mother's strangeness and indifference. His father had also threatened him with the worst if he didn't ask the judge to return home.

The juvenile court judge went even further and suspended the family weekends for good. Stéphane only saw his parents for a short time each quarter, at the social center, accompanied by a psychologist who sometimes had to restrain this over-invasive and sometimes threatening father. To his great relief, Stéphane never returned to his parents' home again, until that last summer when he had to return to the house of his nightmares to sort through objects and papers, and reconnect with his memories.

Stéphane continues to explain the latest events.

"I didn't want to inherit from my father, I didn't get along with my parents, I didn't feel any friendship for them. My mother made me, but in a way, she's not my mother. For one thing, she didn't raise me. There's no emotional bond. When I was a baby, she was far too ill to take care of me, so my sister did until I was placed in care. And then all my difficulties, the feeling of insecurity I always feel everywhere, it's because of them. They were a danger to me, I was suspicious of everything, I was on the alert all the time, and I've always been. Ever since I was a child, I've always thought the worst, and my parents are the cause of all my problems. So life's no fun, it's ingrained in my head. When I was younger, I was always tense, never serene. I still can't control that stress. Besides, I was a bit ashamed of the way they were. If my father scared me, it was my mother who shocked me the most. I changed my surname three times. As a baby, I bore my mother's married name, but then she divorced me and had her paternity annulled. I then took her maiden name. Then my father recognized me and I took his name. During a visit with the psychologist, he explained that he wasn't my father, but that he had recognized me to get my mother to agree to marry him. She had probably hoped that a new situation as a married woman with a husband who had declared himself my father would give her a better chance of getting me back.

The only time I had peace of mind was when I went far away on vacation with my host family. Far from being an exile, these holiday trips were a relief: there was no risk of running into them. During these trips, my host parents always had me write and send a postcard to my birth parents.

There were times when my parents were shopping in the department store where I worked, and they would watch me from a distance, observing me from behind the shelves, but they remained discreet and didn't try to approach me. A year ago, they came back and, in front of the customers and my colleagues, insisted on giving me an envelope full of money. At first I refused, but to avoid public scandal, shame and trouble at work - I was afraid my father would end up getting very angry - I finally agreed. That evening, with a colleague who sometimes helped me, I went to their house to return the money, which was a very large sum. My father was not at all happy. I didn't want anything from them. The things in the house, the inheritance, it's the same thing, I didn't want any of it, I could see too much that it came from them.

Somehow, they must have suffered from the fact that they had been found incapable of looking after me, that I had been taken away from them. They didn't choose to be mentally ill, and I understand them a little, but I've been through too much with them. I try to weigh up the pros and cons, not to see everything only in negative terms. That's what I think, because I've been through this or that, but they've been through things differently. Managing the estate and inheritance, moving back into the house, brought back too many bad memories. And then, I also saw some strange things that surprised me. When I was putting away my father's things, I came across the postcards my host family used to send me when we went on trips: my father had kept them all.

My foster parents were very present throughout this period after my father's death. They thought it would be good for me to keep something of his. I chose to take his car and sold my scooter. It'll be easier to get to work.

But I don't want to carry on the family name. I asked my foster parents if they would adopt me. They agreed. I'll be able to change my surname and finally bear their name. After the name of a stranger, after that of my mother, after that of my mother's husband, I'm going to bear a fourth family name, and that's the name I want to have. True parents aren't the ones who gave birth to you, but the ones who love you and invest themselves in you."

When he came back to see me, I asked Stéphane to read him this text, which is a transcription of everything I've understood and heard over the twenty years I've known him on a more or less regular basis. He accepted, listened attentively to my reading, which I tried to make as neutral as possible, and then said:

"It was a pleasure to hear my story."

Stéphane only stayed with his mother for two months, between his second and fourth months. This period of emotional isolation had dramatic consequences, the after-effects of which Stéphane still retains, despite intensive psychic resuscitation care, long-term placement in a loving foster family who adopted him when he came of age, prolonged psychological care and a drastic reduction in his parents' visiting rights. He continues to suffer from disabling anxiety disorders and reduced social and relational efficiency. Should we consider Stéphane resilient?

Resilient? *Resilience.* A fashionable concept that has its limits and requires certain conditions to be applied to children in the child welfare system.

This is the definition of resilience: a stress applied to an object deforms it, but once the action is complete, the object returns to its initial state.

Resilience is a term from the physical sciences, concerning the resistance of materials and the study of breaking points. This notion was transposed to the psychic domain by Boris Cyrulnik - a lover of oxymorons - who popularized the concept of psychic resilience with real success. In the very first pages of his book *Un merveilleux malheur*[45], he writes: "Where we marvel at meeting children who triumph over their misfortunes." It's true that, beyond the traumas they have endured, some children retain a potential for development and recovery that is sometimes astounding. Boris Cyrulnik's theory is based on observations of children who have developed unimaginable talents and recovered from traumas that are difficult to recover from. Knowing that children so painfully affected by bereavement, war, abuse

---

45. CYRULNIK (Boris), *Un merveilleux malheur*, Paris, Odile Jacob, 1999.

or serious illness can get on with their lives encourages us not to be petrified by the face of horror, but to accompany and support them in their desire to live again.

But this concept, poorly assimilated in child protection circles, from judges to politicians, from child psychiatrists to educators, sometimes justifies a wait-and-see attitude in intervention decisions, which are then taken too late, with irreversible consequences for the children.

Indeed, his readers have mainly retained only this aspect of his demonstration: the possible restoration of the subject, as Boris Cyrulnik's own happy personality testifies. As a result of this truncated reading, professionals sometimes imagine that children have become stainless, capable of resisting anything, because they are resilient by definition, and that with a being in the making, so young, so malleable, there's no hurry...

Yet Boris Cyrulnik is very clear. Resilience requires a condition in order to be exercised. He points out that a child must have known a loving environment, "good enough" as Winnicott would have said, and affective security throughout his or her first year at least, in order to acquire a capacity for resilience: "There is a profile of traumatized children who have the aptitude for resilience, those who have acquired the 'primitive trust' between zero and twelve months: I was loved, therefore I am lovable, therefore I keep the hope of meeting someone who will help me resume my development."[46]

---

46. CYRULNIK (Boris), "Il y a une vie après l'horreur. Interview", collected by BOUKHARI (Sophie), *Le Courrier de l'Unesco*, November 2001.

"Grown Ups are Really Stupid"

At the very end of his book, Boris Cyrulnik concludes that resilience also has a cost for the subject. "Resilience is more than resisting, it's also learning to live. Unfortunately, it's expensive", he says, having taken decades to be able to talk about his story as a child, brutally orphaned by the deportation of his parents to the Nazi extermination camps. And it's likely that it was the long process of constructing his theory of resilience that enabled him to break his lease on the traumas of the past. Resilience is an intellectual theory that he developed and whose elaboration nourished his own resilience. But before that, he was lucky enough to have known the love of his parents. His zest for life is certainly their legacy.

In *Histoire d'une vie (Story of a Life)*[47], the writer Aharon Appelfeld, whose dramatic story is similar, recounts with infinite tenderness the jubilant wonder of his childhood with his parents and their delicate affection, right up to the point of tragedy. "Of those distant, buried days, no words remain in my memory, only my mother's looks. They contained so much gentleness and care for me that I can still feel them today."

A possible resilience is subject to one condition - having received a prior affective endowment, i.e. having had the positive experience of trust in others - but will also presuppose a significant psychic expenditure throughout the subject's reconstruction. This second process requires quality emotional support and a great deal of time. "For many years, I was plunged into an amnesiac sleep [...] This book is not a summary, but rather an attempt, a desperate

------

47. APPELFELD (Aharon), *Story of a Life*, Paris, Éditions de l'Olivier, 2004.

effort to connect the different strata of my life to their roots," says Aharon Appelfeld, fifty years after the tragedy.

The very young children in this book, such as Kévin, Amélie, Cathy, Yannick, Karl, Simon, Léna and Martin, were not so lucky as to have been pampered, loved and surrounded during their first months of life. They had no experience and therefore no confidence in their ability to be loved. Their resilience was weak. That's why it was so difficult for them to rely on the professionals who offered them their presence and attention.

You don't have to wait until a child has been destroyed by unacceptable living conditions to remove him or her from a traumatic family environment. Too much is too late.

The younger the child, the more serious and irreversible the damage.

When the child's personality and emotional security have been severely damaged, separation will be no less avoidable, but will be an additional ordeal.

Some very young children admitted to the nursery have suffered such emotional deprivation that they experience even the most respectful gestures of human care as an aggression. This is what makes their care so complicated. They appear to be persecuted by the adult, destroying any bonds they may form by interpreting them as threats. Previous experience of chaos casts its shadow over the environment, however reassuring. Some fall into madness. How do you grow up in these conditions?

It would then be tempting to conclude that it was the placement that was toxic or harmful, whereas it was its late nature that led to the disintegration of the child's personality.

Re-feeding a severely malnourished hunger striker too quickly and too late can lead to death. But you don't draw the conclusion that eating is dangerous.

For a child already shaken by previous ordeals, placement will represent a real obstacle course, and he'll have to become a top-level mental athlete to cope with the events that follow. He'll need to find the resources within himself to adapt to a foster family, to cope with possible changes of foster home during childhood, to deal with his family's history and to confront the personalities of his parents, who are sometimes still very much present. Living in society with the intimate secret of having been removed from your parents' care, without being able to rely on their pride, is painful. This event will always have an impact on school integration and friendships during childhood, and on love choices and self-confidence in adolescence and adulthood.

In 1840, Dr. Montfalcon was unaware of the theory of resilience. But he was already aware of the emotional and human cost of not having benefited from the respectful affection of his parents: "The injustice of the world ceaselessly blames the foundling for a fault that is not his, for a misfortune that is not his work; his birth is often thrown at him like the bloodiest of insults; it becomes for him a sign of reprobation that nothing can henceforth erase. Without family, without friends, fed by public pity which ceaselessly haggles over the bread it offers him, and rejected by all, the orphan often passes unknown and despised on this earth, like a shipwrecked traveler on a foreign beach."[48]

---

48. TERME and MONTFALCON, *op. cit.*

Today, the quality of care and support for children in the child welfare system has greatly improved. Children are no longer stigmatized by society as being on welfare.

While ordinary children who have experienced tragedy can find enough resources within themselves to rely on reliable adults other than their family environment, children entrusted to child protection services have neither this opportunity nor this chance.

These children need meticulous support if they are to mobilize their resilience, weakened by previous deleterious experiences.

Affection and goodwill are not enough on their own, and must be applied in a structured way, subject to a very detailed analysis of the child's needs. The child's needs are sometimes expressed in such subtle ways that this examination requires a seasoned professionalism on the part of all involved, solid training, teamwork based on principles and theoretical benchmarks proven by shared experience, and open questioning of the validity of work choices. This is also the cost of resilience, which requires sufficient resources in terms of trained personnel and time. Improvisation and inadequate responses can be just as destructive as the previous chaos.

Children need to be able to experience what it's like to be told the right things, without being contradicted by vague or contradictory actions. They need to discover that the attention given to them is sincere, without calculation, but without angelism. To feel secure, a child needs containment. In other words, to be surrounded and defended, but also to be bordered and channeled. Containment means both protecting and limiting.

It's also essential to study precisely what his parents can still offer him, and what he needs to be protected from in his relationship with them. It is then possible to build a project adapted to each child's situation, à la carte, with very different configurations from one child to another, from one family to another.

14.

DAVID IS LOOKING FOR A FAMILY

Are you sure you're your child's only parents?

"Quæ lactat, mater magis quam quæ genuit."[49]

David lived only a short time with his father, who returned to Africa without recognizing him. His mother, too, disappeared one cold, cruel night of partying. Leaving a very drunken party with "friends", she collapsed, dead drunk, on a frozen sidewalk, waiting for a hypothetical cab that never came. Her sobered-up "friends" discovered her in the morning, too late. They also found David asleep, fortunately forgotten in a corner of the apartment. A vague godmother of his mother's, from who knows where, took him in and protected him from a couple who, having neither children nor scruples, were ready to adopt him immediately, without formalities, in return for some money to keep

---

49. *Phaedra.* Possible translation: "It is milk that makes a mother more than blood."

the gossips quiet. David ended up in the nursery, where he was entrusted to a foster family.

We got to know each other. The "godmother" who had taken him in agreed to come and tell the little she knew of his story, and bring some poor clothes that David had shared with one of her children. David has no personal effects. The godmother brought a crumpled, blurred photo of a family evening in a dark apartment. One of the women, with barely discernible features, is said to be his mother. She is dancing with an unidentifiable man, photographed from behind. David is in total material and emotional destitution, with no family, no history.

During the interview, he took hold of a game, a kind of one-armed bandit made up of three lines of three images, each of which rotates on its axis. The nine image squares, synchronized on the correct side, can show either a bear's head, an elephant's face or the face of a big, friendly lion, the usual totemic animals of childhood. But as with the reconstruction of a composite portrait, it's possible to build a composite figure: bear forehead, elephant trunk, lion jowls or any other imaginable combination until the anthropomorphic face is completely destructured: right lion ear, left elephant ear, right bear eye, left lion eye, and so on. At the tender age of four, David quickly understands how this game works, but turns it on its head. As we evoke the various attachment figures he has encountered in his short life - his father, his mother, the godmother, the foster family where he has been living for the past few days - David rolls the images around, in total disorder, then ends up stabilizing each roll in between, constructing a hybrid figure of eighteen pieces of half-eye, half-ear, half-mouth, a shattered, incomprehensible and blurred kaleidoscopic image that makes you dizzy and dizzy. In the casino of life, the one-armed bandit didn't spoil him. David is in disarray, in search of stable attachments and an identity.

We take a look at David's arrival in his foster home. At his childminder's, he asks where "his dead mother" is. He also asks every man he meets - friend, neighbor, letter carrier, teacher - if he wants to be his daddy. He also asked his nanny to write on a slate his first name, *David*, then her first name, then her husband's first name. To complete this declaration and request for love, David then explains:

"You're not my family, but I live in your house."

For several days, he remained glued to her, never letting more than a meter separate them. When he arrived without a cuddly toy, he adopted the first cushion he could find before being offered a real one. His childminder had bought him some clothes and a small toiletry kit, but she became a little annoyed when he refused to use the toothbrush. David had placed it carefully on his bedside table as a precious gift: you don't wash with a gift. He admires it on the shelf where it's displayed, but refuses to use it in his games.

Children have the ability to help you understand complex psychological concepts in a simple way, and you'll often find yourself at a loss when you read a dry psychology textbook.

So it is with the notions of identity formation, identification and affiliation. Who am I, who have I chosen to be like, and who do I grant the right to love me? Children can show us this mysterious and secret alchemy, this intimate and occult combinatorial process, by revealing how they compose and construct their own parental images, and thus their identity. These questions are particularly relevant to children without families and children with multiple parentage. Multiple filiation means having several fathers or mothers. The most frequent situation is that of a child living in a blended family - following a new union after a bereavement or separation - where he or she has to structure themselves with more than two parental images. This is also the case for a child who has been adopted or is living with a foster family, or a child born of donor insemination or living with a homosexual couple. But it's also the case for a child raised by a single parent who doesn't know who fathered him or her, or who was born to a surrogate mother. The diversity of these situations shows that this picture, which at first glance seems very particular, is in fact very widespread. This is the general situation of children whose biological filiation does not cover the reality of an emotional or nurturing parental couple. Children do not choose the lives of their parents, and family laws are always one step behind changing mores. The question is not to pass judgment on the merits or otherwise of these life choices, but to understand how children adapt to them. Because, in reality, this is a question for every child, and has been for every one of us.

Freud, in his short four-page article of 1909, *The Family Story of the Neurotic*[50], wrote that at a time in childhood when the child is beginning to detach itself from its parents, "phantasmatic activity takes on the task of getting rid of the parents, now disdained, and substituting others for them". But with his genius for observation, he adds that "these new, more distinguished parents are endowed with traits

---

50. FREUD (Sigmund), "Le roman familial des névrosés" (1909), in *Névrose, psychose et perversion*, Paris, PUF, 1973, pp. 157-160.

"Grown Ups are Really Stupid"

that all derive from real memories of the true parents". In this Freudian elaboration, the child constructs imaginary fantasy parents with certain "traits" of his or her real parents. Two years later, Carl Gustav Jung, in *Metamorphoses and Symbols of the Libido,* introduced the term *imago* parental, which can be defined as the imaginary construction of a parent, a representation that is highly emotionally charged. Following on from these two authors, we can define the parental imago as an imaginary representation of the parent, "reconditioned" by the child through the prism of his or her passionate experiences and affective motions.

In the case of children with multiple filiation, the child not only transforms a single maternal figure and a single paternal figure, but constructs his maternal and paternal imagos from several parental figures that he superimposes and merges around a nodal point, common to these multiple but stacked images. His parental imagos are thus colored by all his experiences of attachment to the successive parental figures who were vital to him at some point in his existence. The child identifies a common trait in each parental representation, and "staples" the "photos" together at that precise point. This enables him to compose a single image from several representations, and build the story of his identity in several layers. This layer traces the superimposition of his successive or simultaneous affiliations with parental figures, fathers, mothers and other key figures from his childhood, with whom he wanted to be loved. This psychic work seeks to build a link for the subject, reminiscent of the symbolic filiation defined by Guyotat[51],

---

51. GUYOTAT (Jean), "Traumatisme et lien de filiation", *Dialogue,* no. 168, Érès, February 2005.

between blood filiation - that of DNA tests - and instituted filiation - that enshrined in law.

No imaginary stabilization of parental imagos without this assembly work, which goes beyond the simple question of the search for origins. There can be no adhesion to a foster or adoptive family, no emotional stability in a blended family, without the collage work reminiscent of this pictorial technique. This is not always done without internal conflict. When children are unable to condense their attachment figures in this way, usually because of concealment, lies or adult conflicts, their imagination wanders in search of unstable identifications that absorb all their vital and intellectual energy and parasitize all their affective bonds, as David showed with his one-armed bandit. On the contrary, when these images are assembled and stabilized, the child can go on with his life without being persecuted by this black hole of identifications.

It's necessary to present a few examples to describe various resolutions to this question, each one personal to a child. As we've already said, each child is a unique author and actor in his or her own original scenario.

Jules shows an ambivalent affiliation with her childminder.

Seven-year-old Jules had a parental role in his family, competently looking after his sister, calming her down, reassuring her when his mother, exasperated by the little girl's crying, threatened to smash her into the wall.

He has just been taken in by a foster family, where he refuses to eat what his nanny gives him, or only eats when forced to. He refused to eat the copious and varied breakfast offered to him by his kindergarten assistant, who was full of good intentions, having been informed of the food deprivation Jules had suffered. He scorned the feast, contenting himself with a glass of cold milk and a handful of cereals. The same restrictions apply to lunch and dinner, to the annoyance of his hostess, who scolds him more or less at the end of each meal, angry that he's not eating all the good things she's prepared for him. One evening, when there wasn't enough time to eat together, the childminder gave her free rein to draw up the menu for his dinner. Jules can help himself to whatever he likes. And so, freed from the constraint of feeding himself for his own good, he eats for his own pleasure. His appetite for food is amazing, which surprises the whole family. The kindergarten assistant observes this behaviour, is amused by it and opens up to Jules about it:

"Ah! I'm glad you've finally allowed yourself to taste all the goodies on offer!"

Jules, as soon as he hears these words of compliment - the first congratulations at the end of a meal! - he rushes off to vomit his dinner without being able to explain why. This happened at a time when Jules was adapting better and better to the family, allowing himself to make emotional demands on his foster parents, and beginning to confide in them about his difficult life before.

The solution to this riddle came from his mother. She incidentally recounted how she used to give her son a glass of cold milk and some cereal in the morning. Jules, mindful of his mother's psychological fragility and protective of her as he was of his little sister, insisted on remaining faithful to her diet, unconsciously continuing to be her anxious protector. But as he became more and more relaxed in the foster home, his concern for his mother slackened, until this betrayal in the womb. He didn't realize it until afterwards, when he was complimented by the foster carer. His sudden appetite had reflected the well-being of his budding affiliation with this family, but had been a betrayal of his duty of worried devotion to his mother. It was too much! Anguish for his fragile mother, for a moment forgotten, overwhelmed him, and the proof of this emotional laxity, this meal of forgetfulness, had to be erased.

Another example is Jacques' conflict of affiliation with his benevolent stepmother.

Eight-year-old Jacques comes for a consultation with his father and stepmother. His stepmother explains that "there's nothing going on between Jacques and her". His father confirms the relationship difficulties that only exist between this woman and this child: everything else is fine. Jacques refuses his stepmother's gestures of affection, regarding her as a stranger, and refuses to listen to her or carry out any instructions at home. He either ignores her or is insolent. His stepmother is deeply hurt that Jules doesn't love her.

Jacques explains that it's absolutely no problem for him not to love his mother-in-law, since he ignores her and she doesn't exist for him.

My answer to this family is that feelings don't impose themselves and remain a mystery. I'm all too aware that some uprooted children always live in exile, nostalgic for their lost parents - sometimes lost in the imagination following a separation - and will never feel at home in a new family (blended, foster, adopted) that they consider foreign or illegitimate. Or at least, they'll have ambivalent, mixed feelings. Jacques doesn't want to build any bridges between mother and mother-in-law figures.

If filiation is written, affiliation cannot be ordered.

A few weeks later, however, Jacques tells me that he'd had enough of being in conflict with Marie, his mother-in-law, and that he'd tried to respond less, to listen better, and that "now she's become nice. We used to quarrel all the time, but not any more".

Seven-year-old Ludovic was rushed to the emergency room by his parents because he said he wanted to leave the family, run away from home, join the clouds and die. In the kitchen, he put his money where his mouth was, grabbing sharp knives and threatening to "kill himself". He can no longer fall asleep at night.

For the past few weeks, Ludovic had been taking everything the wrong way, both at home and at school. He'd become irascible and short-tempered, which wasn't like him. A complete turnaround. He even told his mother that he hated her and didn't like the family.

Ludovic explains that about a year ago, while looking at vacation photos, he was surprised that he didn't have the same hair color as his brothers and sisters:

"My brother and I weren't the same, we don't have the same hair and we don't look at all alike."

A question then came to him about his parentage, and he wondered if he wasn't an adopted child. It was an irrelevant question, but one that nagged at him for months, and one that would come as a great surprise to his parents when they learned of it during this recent consultation.

Three weeks before this interview, Ludovic, on a Sunday family walk, fell into a ditch, left his shoe stuck in the mud, was reprimanded by his father and gently mocked by the rest of the family, amused by this burlesque episode. Ludovic felt ridiculed and scorned. It was the shovelful of mud that made the trough overflow. He interpreted this misfortune and disgrace as the ultimate proof of his strangeness to this family. He was indeed an adopted child. What followed was an anxious, violent and suicidal episode in the context of a feeling of emotional disarray. In the future, Ludovic will certainly have to find points of identification with his family other than hair color, which seems to be well on the way.

However, not all affiliations are conflictual, as Bryan, Benoît and Tatiana show us, who manage to bring their multiple parents together.

On my advice, five-year-old Bryan is informed that "Dad", the man who raised him and whom he loves, is his step-father. Logically, Bryan immediately asks who his father is. His mother agrees to contact his "ex", who promptly turns up to meet her son - it's never too late to introduce yourself to your offspring!...

It's evening in the apartment, and Mother and "Dad", a tad anxious about the possible effects of this meeting on Bryan, are milling around waiting for "Dad" to pay them a solemn visit. Every few minutes, Bryan lifts the window curtain to look out into the street. Suddenly, he sees a delivery van slow down and park on the other side of the street. A man gets out and crosses the street. The doorbell rings and Bryan meets his father.

"It went well," his mother confirms at the next appointment. Bryan then explains:

"My father has the same truck as Dad", he concluded from his observations of vehicle movements on the street. His father and father-in-law each have a delivery van as a work vehicle. This common mark, this identifying trait, was to become the point of contact for stapling together his two fathers and assembling them into a single image.

Benoît was adopted at the age of two. By the age of six, he was talking freely about his history with his mother, and knew his natural parentage. One day, in a tender moment, he declares to his adoptive mother:

"I'd like your name to be Isabella and my mom from Colombia's name to be Catherine."

By swapping first names in this way, he declares how much he would have liked to have been born to this woman without denying his birth mother, blending their destinies and his own in a peaceful way.

Tatiana, a cheerful four-year-old girl, was also adopted a year ago. She sums up the need for coexistence and introjection of her natural and adoptive parents in a little refrain that she sings often. The perfection and conciseness of her formula are extraordinary:

"I have two moms,
one in the belly
and one in the heart...
I have two moms..."

It is Tatiana who brings her parents together and carries them within her.

The success of a foster placement or adoption is generally confirmed and guaranteed by observing the child's non-conflictual signs of affiliation with his or her surrogate parents, and by pinpointing the point at which parental images come together.

Camille shows us how these complex issues can be addressed through psychotherapy.

Five-year-old Camille was abandoned shortly after birth in a small house in an Asian village square on a market day. The circumstances of the time and place of this abandonment demonstrate her mother's determination that the baby should soon be found and taken in. She was adopted a few months later.

Her adoptive mother came to see me with her a year ago, due to a constant daydreaming that never allowed her daughter to get on with what she was doing, and which was causing major difficulties in adapting to the classroom. The situation has improved considerably since then. Today, Camille is doing well, but her original question, now more circumscribed, limited to the time of our interviews and reappearing incidentally with her adoptive mother, is still present. How to live with two moms, how to make them coexist.

Camille systematically draws two houses side by side.

At our first meeting, she dramatized her abandonment by her birth mother and her adoptive mother's lack of a child, and drew me two rudimentary squares: an empty house next to a house containing an infant on the floor. This is what she explained to me. A staging of her abandonment and discovery. But also a full mother and an empty mother. It was a very sad drawing, drawn in a single color, without any embellishment, bringing these two women together in the pain of an impossible childbirth.

Later, she asked her adoptive mother:

"My birth mother, what's her name? I know because I know her, I know her name, but it's a secret."

It wasn't a question but a riddle, and Camille pretended to wait for the answer:

"It starts with a D (she has a surname beginning with D). It's like Durand (her surname), but it's not Durand and then her name is Elisabeth."

Camille tries to match the two maternal images by name, identical in her riddle, but the collage seems unstable.

The question, far from being exhausted, comes up again and again. Camille asks:

"Did you understand when my mother spoke to you in Chinese? I understood because I speak Chinese," she adds, inventing an imaginary meeting between the two mothers, who remain irremediably strangers to each other in her narrative. Or Camille may speak to her mother with a curious accent that purports to be foreign, explaining that she doesn't speak French. In these speeches, she is the only one who knows her two mother tongues, but they are languages that are foreign to each other. Camille sees herself as the common link between these two women, definitively separated by the language barrier, and so cannot yet merge them into a single imago.

This week, Camille again drew two tall identical houses side by side on the same sheet of paper. They're beautifully drawn houses. She writes the letter D on one and the letter T on the other. A cat is asleep on a bed on the second floor of one of them. She comments:

"The cat changes houses all the time."

But she also draws a girl with multicolored hair, because "it's fashionable and she wants to," she tells me. A true rainbow, which undoubtedly marks the beginning of a solution for blending the colors of her parentage.

So we still have some psychotherapeutic work to do together, even though everything seems to be going well in class, at home and in her leisure activities. Camille has

14. David is Looking for a Family

expressed a strong desire to continue talking with me. His mother, who understands this very well, gives me every latitude and freedom, but I would be very embarrassed, in front of other less astute parents, to have to explain that their child should continue to talk when he seems "cured".

I remember, in particular, a little Inès, aged six or seven, adopted as a baby by parents who were nevertheless charming, but who understood nothing of their daughter's need to come back regularly to see me to talk about her multiple parental imagos, something she wouldn't allow herself to do in front of them. They had decided, on the strength of their daughter's apparently recovered mental health, to cut short the interviews. Inès negotiated "one more appointment" with her mother. When she came back the following week for the last one, she gave me a bag of pebbles, small pebbles she'd picked up in a stream on her last vacation, to pay me, she explained, for all the sessions she'd no longer be coming to. They still clutter my drawer many years later.

Great care must be taken to honor and respect the images of parents that every child carries and treasures, more intimate and secret than his or her genes, beneficial or terrifying, that no separation can make disappear, that no words can ever erase, something that many adults would like to forget.

15.

Adriano, the Alchemist

Caring: nurturing and educating

Where the reader discovers the inner workings of child psychotherapy. The aim of a treatment is to reorganize the child's master signifiers, i.e. the few words and their imaginary representations that structure him and determine his position in the family and in the world. It's a game of push-pull or tease, where you have to figure out how to restore fluidity to a frozen system, by moving one square piece after another. The game is stuck, but you're asked to give it movement again, after everyone else has tried everything else. You're not allowed a screwdriver. It's just a game of sleight of hand with signifiers.

In Adriano's case, there were nine square pieces for nine squares. No empty square, system blocked. There were two "mom" squares, two "home" squares, two "patronymic" squares, one "secret" square, two "Adriano" squares, i.e. M M R R P P S A A.

My work consisted of seeing him a dozen times, expressing my interest in his graphic productions and making a technical error on the first meeting, which he didn't hold against me. I also scrupulously noted down the sequence of moving pieces, as in chess.

This work also had the opposite effect to that hoped for: too much fluidity.

Seven-year-old Adriano took charge right from the word go. He showed me the path to follow and the goal to reach.

On a half-sheet of paper, in the left half, he draws a rather lanky, feminine-looking figure with long hair. In the space on the right, he inscribes the word "*Mom*" in a cartouche.

- Who's this mom you've drawn?

- It's Valerie! (The childminder who accompanied him introduced herself by that name).

He turns this small sheet over and, on the back, depicts another character, this one large, his mouth distorted by a sneer. He writes: "Beauty and the beast". I ask him what it means:

"It's a beast," he says, taking the outstretched paper between his two hands and bringing it up to my eyes as if he were presenting me with a protest banner. And I see through the paper the two superimposed characters, the "mother" and the "beast". Both sides irreconcilable.

Flabbergasted, I ask him if I can make a photocopy of his drawings to remind me. My mistake: I photocopied the obverse and reverse on the same side. The resulting copy has the two designs one on top of the other. The back-to-back became a side-by-side. Mother Beauty and Mother Beast on the same page. Adriano was quick to appropriate this new representation, which he conscientiously began to colorize like an old film in need of remastering. The violent light of the photocopier has captured the name of the cartridge through the paper[52]: each of the two characters is given a "maman". Adriano thus has two moms, one of whom is clearly more relatable than the other in his eyes.

Adriano has already told me everything, explained everything, shown everything, and I shouldn't have to listen to any of the interfering elements that are bound to interfere with the work ahead. If he is to continue growing, he will have to find something in common - a unary trait, as the Lacanians would say - between these two women. He loves one of them, allowing himself to exercise a daily tyranny over her, knowing her benevolence and bonhomie. He would also like to be loved by the other, who doesn't come to see him, forgets him. He complains openly.

Second session, it gets complicated!

This time, it's not the doubling of mothers he's showing me, but the doubling of residences. First drawing, a fortified castle, bristling with bars and railings. Two tiny loopholes with curtains. In one of the towers, the prison.

Second drawing, a pretty house, a flower garden. The parents have stored lots of presents for the children in the attic. From a large window with raised curtains, a young girl waves goodbye. She's named after his sister. He writes: "the house of Mr. and Mrs. Faucon, of Caroline and Johnny", an imaginary family, who are enrolling him and his sister in their foster home. He adds on the sheet, as if it were a school assignment, "parents' signature" and explains to me:

"Valérie will sign."

But he signs the drawing with his own surname.

---

52. Without realizing it at the time, I had created a Möbius strip from the two drawings, in the Lacanian sense of the term.

Dual mothers, dual residences, dual surnames. Six squares.

I'm familiar with the psychic work of children who, not living with their parents or having several parents, need to build a stable representation of what a mother or father is. Whether they're adopted, living with a foster family, in a blended family or born through gamete donation, they take a piece of this, a piece of that, from each other, and cobble together their maternal and paternal "imagos", like others make genetically modified organisms. Every "ordinary" child does this in an imaginary way, but others have this obligation to build it for real, with their imagination, inspired by the crumbs of reality. Adriano, a foster child, could have been, should have been, in this usual, let's say classic, dimension. Two mothers, two homes, two surnames. But the configuration turns out to be far more complicated: an affectionate mother and a less-than-presentable mother, a dapper house with an attic full of treasures and a fortress in a remote province, a name that won't go away.

I should have been wary of the monstrous mother figure that poked its nose through the paper and of this other, even more mysterious figure, locked away far away behind heavy walls and bars. A nameless shadow. Secret room, seven squares.

I am given information about this child's story. Adriano, born prematurely, was hospitalized for eight weeks before being allowed to return home to his parents. They were imprisoned two months later, the father being one of the instigators of a vast network of paedophiles who prostituted their own children. Adriano's siblings were among the victims of this appalling affair. The children were all taken into care, Adriano with them. He was the youngest. Staying at home for only a short time, he escaped the horrors that had been going on for years. The chance of his young age protected him from this infamy, but as he was not himself a direct victim of his parents, they retained their parental authority over him[53]. An incredible act of judicial perjury, even though this right was withdrawn for all siblings. The father was sentenced to several decades in prison.

Yet I had a fleeting intuition that it would have been better not to know. The sheets of drawing paper, colored, light and translucent, suddenly took on a grayish hue and the weight of lead.

How will Adriano negotiate this terrible inheritance? How will he achieve the alloy of gold and lead, the vile metal, between the parental imagos of his natural family and his foster family? I don't know. What I do know is that I'm going to have to go down the lead mine with him, to face the fear of the dark, the claustrophobia, the pitfalls, the ghosts, the spectres, the secrets of shame, the

---

53. Aeschines, 390-314, who is said to have been a disciple of Socrates, wrote: "The legislator then speaks of serious offences, but which, no doubt, are committed in the city: for our ancients only passed laws to oppose dykes to real excesses. The law therefore states, in no uncertain terms, that if a father, brother, uncle, guardian or anyone else who has authority over a child sells it and gives it over to the pleasures of others, it is not the child who can be accused, but the person who bought it and the person who sold it; one, it says, for having bought it, and the other for having sold it: it has established the same penalties against both. Twenty-four centuries ago, Athenian law was more protective of children than it is today! Discours contre Timaque", in *Œuvres complètes de Démosthène et d'Eschine*, translated from the Greek by Abbé Auger, Paris, Verdière, 1820.

15. Adriano, the Alchemist

monsters and the nightmares that haunt this dark and horrific family history.

I don't know what to do with my teasing game anymore.

Next session.

"Adriano has had a motorcycle accident," he explains. He draws the overturned motorcycle, the ambulance that takes Adriano from the village where he lives to the town where I work. Adriano is lying on a hospital bed. His left arm and leg are in plaster. On the right, his limbs are unharmed. This is a hemi-injured body, one half healthy, the other half fractured, but healed. Always this double or divided image. Adriano, two squares, for a total of nine. For nine squares. System blocked.

Until then, evocations of his natural family were always carefully separated in his drawings from those of his foster family. Obverse and reverse, successive, or above and below, but never confused. This time, Adriano succeeds in constructing a divided representation of himself, half healthy right, half injured left, but in which his bodily unity is preserved. Reduced to eight squares, perhaps less, over nine squares. A fluid, floating, even unstable system.

Has he finally found a way out?

An accident victim, he manages to incorporate his family of "broken arms" into a body that retains its integrity despite the family cataclysm. He now sees himself as a fully-fledged member of his foster family. But he keeps a piece of his natural family grafted onto his body, almost like a mummified receiver. Surgical sequestration in his body image, judicial sequestration in his life. It's a part of him, diseased and carefully isolated from the rest of his body, a residual witness to another life, in sanitary quarantine inside himself. This family wound is only visible on the X-ray produced by the photocopier. But his host family knows about it, and takes good care of Adriano and his wound, with delicacy and discretion, taking him to the "shrink doctor" in town.

The last session?

"[...] I don't feel like drawing anymore, I want to play dominoes [...]" and we played, mute as carp. Only the sharp clacking of the wooden pieces placed one by one on the table punctuated our exchange in a soothed silence.

Adriano didn't come back for a few months.

This confused, parasitic, distracted, worried little boy, who couldn't maintain his attention either at school or at his childminder's, had changed completely. Suddenly freed from the burden of having to carry the family history he'd been dragging around like a convict with a ball and chain, he became light, carefree and hyperactive! His ADD was still there, but very different. From leaden he had become an elusive zebrafish. But joyful, inventive, effervescent, sparkling.

The party had its downside. His school results became disastrous, and he stopped doing any work at all. He was disrespectful of all rules and disregardful of others, whether with his carer or outside. He was a child who let himself be guided only by his own pleasure. Intense. Magnificent proof of the total ineffectiveness of all this psychoanalytical nonsense. Education, I tell you! All the rest is poppycock!

Distraught, Valérie, his childminder, came back to see me with him. He and I had a conversation. It boiled down to the fact that I couldn't understand how an intelligent boy like him could jeopardize his social integration and schooling in such a way. And I asked him to come in every month and tell me where he stood on these two issues. Since then, I've been happy to receive him, and his conversation is pleasant. He has a lively, inquisitive mind. He teaches me how to make sophisticated paper airplanes, tells me about the trips he's taken with his foster family and a whole lot of other things. His family assistant, whom he refers to as "Mum" here and "Mum" there, confirms that he's doing very well at school, and that no one complains about him any more.

Above all, she understood that, from now on, the darkness of Adriano's family history should no longer interfere with her educational action: she became demanding and firm with him, as with all the children she has educated, her own and those of others. With tenderness, with accuracy and with success.

A child who is very ill in body, in development, in psyche or because of his or her family history, requires care and arouses empathy. How could it be otherwise?

But once the child has been freed from the burden of illness, or the disability has been stabilized, his or her education must continue. This dual obligation of education and care can be difficult to conceive, because at first glance it seems antinomic in such dramatic circumstances.

Care means soothing, repairing, cocooning, protecting, comforting, relieving and sometimes healing. Education, on the other hand, means civilizing, guiding, governing, instructing, even disciplining and policing. What care is meant to give, education is meant to ration. One repairs and brings together, while the other separates and distances. Should we console the grief of a scolded child? How can we reconcile solicitude and high standards?

When a child suffers, parents let their guard down educationally. It's only logical. Parents and caregivers remain delicate and flexible with a child undergoing chemotherapy.

No one would think of punishing a depressed or suicidal child. Parents feel at a loss to reprimand the opposition of a child saddened by their separation, and feel guilty about it. The birth of a young child can sometimes destabilize an older child who feels unloved. Unjustly chastising him for his jealousy only reinforces his delusion: if his parents punish him, it's proof that they prefer the baby.

In these difficult times, parents find themselves forbidden to educate their children. The duty to care, to allow the child to live, takes precedence over the duty to educate, to teach the child how to behave in life.

This was the case for Adriano. His foster mother had devoted herself to protecting him with her wings from the terrifying family history. But Adriano, having finally freed himself from this leaden ball and chain, went from a state of near-depression to a period of jubilant hypomania that overwhelmed Valérie. She was left defending him on his rear, while he escaped forward. Following our conversation, she was reassured by his evolution. She repositioned herself as an educator, allowing herself to make the right demands. Adriano responded well, making a point of being grateful for her concern for him.

This succession of depressive and then jubilant phases is quite common in children's therapy... which is disconcerting for parents. This phenomenon is reinforced by the trust - to trust is to entrust - that parents place in the therapist, delegating to him - for a time and wrongly, but can we blame them - their educational responsibilities. When the child gets better and regains an unusual vigor, the parents are sometimes surprised to have to take over the reins after having let go of the reins, worried as they were about the child's survival or his appetite for life.

16.

B., the Telephone Man

The misunderstanding of the encounter

This is the last story. I started it a long time ago. The words kept adding up, but it just wouldn't take. My ambition was to let the reader experience the power of babies' emotions, but nothing worked. It wasn't a blank page, just words lined up one after the other. But they were empty words. It was as cold as the boiler operating instructions: "The mixing valve features an electrothermal servo-control device with a fluid expansion system with heating resistance."

I've given up.

The situation was still clear in my memory. Our department head provided me with observations and notes. I read and re-read the file. A colleague told me the story again. I knew it all by heart.

The words wouldn't come.

It takes a flash to build a story. One word meets another and an image is formed. No word wanted to connect with another. And the story was not told well.

Suddenly, the obvious became clear: this was the story of a mother and a child, and it wasn't going well. It hadn't begun at all: they'd never met! How do you talk about nothing? How to talk about the story that didn't exist between them? There was nothing to talk about. A sidereal void.

This baby had just been transferred from the other side of France by court order. The mission assigned to us by the judge was clear: to assess the appropriateness of returning this child to his mother. The whole team at the nursery set out to provide the best possible support for the reunion of mother and child.

The term *"reunion"* is inappropriate: this was a first meeting. This baby had been born by chance at the end of a pregnancy that had gone unnoticed. The mother did not know she was pregnant[54]. The father did not know she was pregnant. The parents separated around the time of the birth. The father left with the child several hundred kilometers to join his own parents. His mother visited him only three times in seven months, and always accompanied by her own parents.

A child who is not in anyone's head is in danger. At the age of four months, he was hospitalized with hematomas in his brain and retinas. He had been "shaken". Several times. Some hematomas were older than others. No one knew

---

54. Today, this is known as pregnancy denial, i.e. the failure to register the physical reality of pregnancy in the woman's psyche, with the logical consequences of this state of affairs: difficulties in investing in the child, which can go as far as denial and infanticide. The various recent cases of frozen babies - Pithiviers 2000, Tours 2006, Albertville 2007, Guingamp 2008, Lasbordes 2011 - have brought this reality back into the media spotlight.

who had done it! For several weeks, the neurosurgeon left him with a tube running down from his skull to his abdomen to relieve the pressure of the fluid compressing his cerebral hemispheres. After eight weeks of treatment, he was placed in a nursery for a few months until a solution could be found. The judge decided not to hand him over to his father, and to evaluate the possibilities with his mother.

The mother honored her visits with regularity and diligence, but there was something not quite right between her and the child. She often seemed "elsewhere", and the baby was quite indifferent to her presence. She did her job as mother, carrying him, feeding him, changing him, taking him for walks, but without any apparent contentment or perceptible affect. The child didn't cry when he saw her, but he didn't smile either. He let himself be taken in and accepted his mother's care, but without visible emotion or shared pleasure. She didn't seek to enter into a relationship with him and remained very distant. There were even times when, as she gazed vaguely into his eyes, his gaze drifted slowly to the side, taking his head with it: he avoided his mother's gaze.

They passed each other, but never met.

She sometimes asked the staff about the child, but it was about his weight, his growth, his meal plan or his vaccinations.

There was no history, and the adventure of living was not written between them. How, under these conditions, could they contemplate returning home? There was nothing to prevent it. The little one would certainly not be in any physical danger around her. But nothing brought them together. It was clear that they couldn't bond. This baby was much less attracted to his mother than to the caregivers. And she seemed almost bored with him. The lack of progress in this sterile weekly routine worried the team.

A relationship that doesn't get off the ground exhausts the partners. This baby was becoming increasingly restless, oppositional and unrewarding. His mother didn't understand him and became impatient. She said she was dissatisfied with the visits and with the baby who cried when she approached. She blamed the restrictive environment in which the meetings took place. Her lawyer pestered the children's judge and criticized the nursery for extending visitation rights. What to tell the judge? What could be done to help them?

We decided to strengthen the framework rather than relax our efforts, by asking the local child psychiatry team to bring in a therapist to accompany each visit, and try to encourage the creation of a bond. Against all odds, the mother agreed, and the work began.

It was a burst of sound that provoked the saving misunderstanding, the meeting of words.

A simple ringing in the corridor. The mother turned her head towards the source of the noise. The baby did the same, which she noticed. They were both looking at the same noise. So she began to tell him about the noise, which turned out to be a hyphen.

"Baptiste! It's the phone ringing! You remembered the phone! Do you remember the phone? When you were far away and I was calling on the phone, do you remember! I used to call every week to ask about you."

Mom was suddenly surprised and moved. She stared intently at her son.

"Mom was thinking about you, you know."

And our colleague adds:

"Baptiste was thinking of you too!"

Baptiste responded with his first real smile. Then he jargonized and suddenly became attentive to the modulations of his mother's voice. That first glance inaugurated a phase of complicity between them, of gradual discovery and new connivance... They had finally met.

Starting with a misunderstanding played out by his mother, to which Baptiste responded. At last, their shared history could be written.

The relationship between Baptiste and his mother gradually grew stronger, with visits always accompanied by our therapist colleague. Baptiste was now very happy to see his mother again, and sad to see her go, which started a virtuous circle between them.

Three months later, the judge logically granted him a definitive return home, with an indication to continue child psychiatric support. Baptiste returned to live with his mother. We were confident. Given the conflictual context of the early days of this placement, we didn't expect to hear from Baptiste. As far as the family was concerned, we were still the bad guys.

A few months later, one of Baptiste's caregivers was shopping in a supermarket. At the bend in the aisle, she came face to face with Baptiste and his mother. These are always delicate situations, as we don't know in advance the parents' wishes or willingness to remember such a troubled period in their lives. Remain discreet, open and respectful.

But it was Baptiste's mother who approached the educator on her own initiative and struck up a conversation, proudly telling her about her son's latest discoveries. Mundane and uninteresting to relate here, but so precious.

The story of Baptiste and his mother, which had a happy ending but could also have resulted in the child's death, raises the question of the desire for a child and the creation of a bond between parent and child.

Despite nine months of absolute physiological dependence, the bond of mutual attraction between mother and child is neither natural nor automatic.

I love horses. My first filly was born unexpectedly one night in April. When I arrived before dawn, this big grasshopper had escaped from her mother and slipped under a fence. She had curled up in the already tall grass of the nearby meadow. It had cooled down. I carried her like a lamb, painstakingly climbed back over the fence and tried to introduce her to her mother, whom I'd locked in a stall. But the little filly tried to feed herself by poking her head under the quarters of an old leather saddle hanging on the partition, while the mare, her udders sore and engorged, refused to let her approach. An impossible reciprocal recognition. A misunderstanding whose unlikely outcome could quickly prove fatal. Worry had overtaken me. It took a lot of patience and cunning to get the wobbly filly to look for nipples elsewhere than under the leather belly of an old saddle, and for the reluctant mare to finally accept her under her. It was all over.

It was the animal ethology model that served as a reference for early work on attachment. As early as 1930, Konrad Lorenz brilliantly demonstrated the phenomenon of imprinting in goslings. You can find amusing old photos on the Internet showing him being followed by a flock of greylag geese, who chose him as their mother goose thanks to the subterfuge of a colored spot he wore on himself when they hatched. The films *Premier envol*

(First Flight) and *Le Peuple migrateur (The Migratory People)*, featuring striking images of a microlight pilot flying accompanied by a flock of geese, were made with animals trained using this method.

These ethological discoveries were transposed to human psychology with great success. In the 1960s, John Bowlby developed the concept of attachment in the mother-child relationship, describing the nature and quality of the emotional bond that develops between child and mother. Some children are more *secure* in their bond with their mother than others - *insecure*. It was not until twenty years later that Mary Ainsworth turned the question on its head with the concept of maternal sensitivity to the child's needs. Some mothers are more sensitive than others in adapting their responses to the child's expressed needs.

While this work had the great advantage of demonstrating that the reciprocal parent-child bond could be a fragile construction - some children are more competent[55] than others in the knotting of the relationship, and some mothers are more sensitive than others in their attention to the child - it abandoned Lorenz's main idea, the notion of imprinting. Interest in studying the quality of the bond overshadowed the question of the processes involved in creating it.

It's a question worth pondering.

On the one hand, how can we explain that a woman could have ignored her pregnancy and abandoned the child she carried? On the other hand, how can we unders-

---

55. The simplest example is the apparent chronological delay in the neurological development of premature babies, who smile later and can cause their parents to despair.

tand how adoptive parents can be amused to see their baby put on their slippers, which they interpret as a sign of belonging. And even more so to hear the adopted baby's grandparents rave about how much he has in common with his parents:

"Oh! He drags his feet like his father."

In order to overcome the apparent contradiction between denial of pregnancy of a biological child and recognition of a child alien to oneself as one's own, it is necessary to break down the constituent elements of the creation of the parental bond.

Around David's story, I developed the concept of affiliation, which we observe in children and which is a concrete expression of the imaginary bond they build with their guardian adults. It's an active process that can be spotted if you pay close attention.

This phenomenon of affiliation has its symmetrical counterpart in parents through imprinting, and what I call kinship.

The parental bond can thus be described as a three-stage construction that overlaps: the desire for a child, the imprint and the matching.

The parental bond is built first and foremost by the desire for a child, based on imaginary and intimate representations of the family and the succession of generations. Pairing is a symbolic bond based on words - "you are my son, you are my daughter" - based on an image, the imprint - "you have this resemblance that brings us together" - much more powerful than the reality of genes and chromosomes.

The curious thing is that they all arise from a misunderstanding. An error of interpretation or perspective, but one that triggers a shared adjustment. The bond between father and child is triggered identically.

The imprint is manifested by the observation of an identity trait in the child, which is not necessarily visual or physical, but can be imaginary, linked to the history of its conception, a date, a dream, a coincidence in existence. This identity trait[56] that the parent recognizes as his or her own has an obvious narcissistic dimension. The imprint is the staple between the imagined child and the child's reality. The commented detail of an ultrasound image is sometimes the first support for this. That's why ultrasound photos of future babies are so popular.

The pairing that immediately follows the imprint is a more socialized process. It is an amplification and a family and social shaping of the initial imprinting process. It is influenced by the personal, family and social context, which can help or hinder the process. The child is then not

56. We note here the imaginary character (of the order of thought and language) of human imprinting, in total contrast to the imaginary character (of the order of a biological reflex signal) of animal imprinting. It's amusing to note that the biological animal model applied to man has nevertheless remained present in the minds of the drafters of the WHO, who advocate good conduct around childbirth, in particular that of skin-to-skin contact, by placing the baby on its mother's belly as soon as it is born. While this practice has been shown to be beneficial for the baby's adaptation to life outside the womb, it has also been suggested that it may encourage the mother's attachment to her child! This idea has also been taken up in recommendations made by the HAS in France. http://www.has-sante.fr/portail/upload/docs/application/pdf/doc.chem.al_22-11-07.pdf

only recognized by his or her parent on a growing series of criteria, but also adopted by the family group.

Each of these stages can have its hazards.

As for the desire for a child, a man or a woman may not want a child at the time it is born, resulting in explicit refusal or denial of pregnancy. But this desire for a child can be so powerful that parents may want to adopt a child who is not of "their blood", as may single people or homosexual couples. A child exists first and foremost in the mind.

In terms of imprinting, this architecture of bonding explains how decisive the first words spoken over a newborn's cradle are, like those spoken by the good and bad fairies in folk tales. That a child will not always be emotionally invested by its mother, and even less often by its father at birth[57]. That adoptive parents can instantly recognize themselves in a child who is not their own, and explain this by a gesture, a look, an attitude, a physical detail or by the child's history.

Ethnology, through the observation of social rituals, reveals the collective expression of individual psychic phenomena. Certain cultures clearly express these stages of imprinting, or refusal of imprinting, and matching. "In very different parts of the world, we find the same ceremony of (false) exposure, mystically protecting the survival of a newborn: among the Mossis of Burkina Faso, if the baby is deemed to be in danger, it is placed on the dump outside the home, like garbage. A neighbor or

---

57. A congenital handicap can represent an insurmountable obstacle to the imprinting phenomenon, which requires narcissistic identification.

passer-by picks it up, and hands it over to the parents with these codified words, inverting the objective relationship of comparse and ascendants: "This newborn is mine (or my slave). Take him, I give him to you to raise." Attested in various West African countries (Côte d'Ivoire, Togo), it can also be found in Singapore: among populations of Malay origin, if a child and its ascendant of the same sex are born on the same day of the week, if they live in the same house, one of the two - the younger - is considered to be in danger; the same applies if the infant is in poor health, or if it is born after a series of children of the same couple who died in infancy. The baby is placed outside in the garbage bin. A woman picks it up and declares: "I recognize the child as mine", places it in the arms of the genitress, enjoining her to raise the young being in the house."[58]

At the beginning of the 20th century, French ethnologist Arnold van Gennep[59] described the mechanism of rites of passage in three phases: separation, the period of margin or isolation, and aggregation. When a child is born, these three phases are represented respectively by the cutting of the cord, medical and childcare care, and the naming of the child, which has the value of kinship. All societies have developed rites around this last stage, such as the *amphi-*

---

58. GUIDETTI (Michèle), LALLEMAND (Suzanne) and MOREL (Marie-France), *Enfances d'ailleurs, d'hier et d'aujourd'hui*, Paris, Armand Colin, coll. "Cursus", 2004, 2nd edition, p. 33.

59. GENNEP (Arnold van), *Les Rites de passage* (1909), Paris, A. et J. Picard, 1981.

dromia[60] of the Greeks or the *lustratio*[61] of the Romans. Today, the social rites of integration of a child into a family and society include recognition by the civil registry, birth announcements and early entry in the family photo album.

These rites demonstrate that the desire for a child, imprinting and matching are purely verbal effects with no biological dimension. A "natural" child must be adopted by its "biological" parents, just like an adopted child or a child born of a gamete donation.

The creation of the parental bond is complex and can therefore prove difficult. But the cultural and social pressure on the duty to give birth is so powerful that few parents allow themselves to express any difficulties they may have in establishing the bond when a child arrives. They should be allowed to talk about it without being stigmatized.

It's surprising how recently these aspects of the parent-child bond have been described. I interpret this as the powerful effect of the cultural injunction to natalize, and the repression of people's unwillingness to have children. Human societies have always been natalist by nature. From Genesis to children's stories, the watchword is "and they had many children". We are programmed to reproduce. But what's good for the human species, renewing generations,

---

60. Literally, "to run around the hearth", i.e. to take the new-born baby on a tour of the house, introducing him or her to the altars of the household gods, including that of the hearth and that of the ancestors.

61. During the *lustratio,* the new child was sprinkled with lustral water using a brandon taken from the domestic hearth. After the ceremony, the child was given his or her name. In ancient times, fire was revered and nurtured as a family deity. When there was no one left to tend the hearth, the family had died out.

doesn't necessarily apply to an individual or a couple: having a child. There are other forms of fertility in life.

This pressure to produce children, whether familial, social or societal, has also changed form. The contemporary era has seen the emergence of the concept of the zero-defect baby, adding quality to the demand for numbers. Parents now have a duty to be good parents. Perhaps that's why you've decided to buy this book.

The parental bond and the filial bond are independent of any biology or predefined family structure.

DNA barcodes are not about to replace the photos of each of us in our family albums.

In Conclusion

At the end of this story, I'm still not sure how much these children have taught me, and of which I've tried to give a few snippets here.

When I started working at the children's home, I quickly realized that all my previous theoretical references - medical, psychiatric, child psychiatric, psychoanalytical - were no longer of any help to me in the face of the catastrophic situation I found myself in. The children were not suffering from the usual psychiatric pathologies for which I had been trained, and I think well trained, by my teachers. These children were severely psychologically polytraumatized, something I'd never encountered before. Their parents had such severe conduct disorders that they didn't fit into any of the mental illness classifications I'd been taught.

So, little by little, I had to reinvent a child clinic and look for other intellectual references, including anthropology, mythology and history, in order to understand parental conduct disorders. I've revealed a few aspects of this in this book. The psychic placenta, the confusion of psyches and affiliation in the child, and imprinting and kinship in the parent, are particularly close to my heart.

But above all, these children taught me not to let myself be hypnotized by the prowling Parque. To look her in the face, measure her full horror and continue on my way.

While children absolutely need adults to understand the seriousness of the tragedies they have experienced, so that they can take the necessary steps to save themselves, they must not remain trapped in the clutches of horror, as if by an evil spell. Children just want to live and grow. It's not a question of forgetting or repressing traumas, but of looking to the future in spite of everything. Children are developing beings, and this dynamic of progress enables them to be reactive if their living conditions change. It's up to adults to take full responsibility. Before it's too late.

I'm one of the last doctors still working in a children's home in France. Soon, there will be none left. So this book was also for me a kind of emergency, a duty to bear witness. Twenty years ago, when I first started working in a children's home, I was stunned by the dramatic state in which some children arrived, even though they had been looked after for months or years by the social services and had been left to be fed to their families. I had hoped that, with time, the justice system, social services and medical services would make progress and stop seeing such desolation, but nothing has really changed. There are still just as many children in such bad shape. Perhaps this book will help raise awareness of the seriousness of their situation, and of the calamitous state of child protection in France, which has been left to lie fallow intellectually since the decentralization laws[62].

Just one figure. While the annual budget for child protection in France exceeds six billion euros[63], the French state spends less than one hundred and fifty thousand euros a year on scientific research programs concerning the future of these children. Less than twenty-five euro cents per child to carry out a hypothetical audit of the quality of their care, and to mobilize improbable research

---

62. In France, after having been a State responsibility, child welfare was departmentalized - under the law of January 6, 1986 - and is now the responsibility of each departmental council. While this organization has brought us closer to the "field", it has also led *ipso facto to* a breakdown in the sharing of practices, the exchange of knowledge and the possible pooling of research resources between departments - a situation condemned to total destitution. Each departmental council has its own policy towards these populations, both in spirit and in budget, with allocations per child that can vary from one to three depending on the department. Far from wishing to defend the centralizing State, it is easy to see that this social policy, which has once again become one-sided and local, despite the fact that it concerns so many children, and which is an excellent indicator of the state of civilization of a community, has caused the organization of child welfare to regress to the system of high and low lords who were in charge of *foundlings* under the Ancien Régime. Fortunately, despite these difficult structural conditions, professionals as a whole are striving to advance the practices and culture of child protection. The Anglo-Saxon countries (USA, Canada, UK) have kept child protection within the bosom of their Ministry of Health, which had been the French situation for the last three centuries.

63. On this subject, read the pertinent conclusion of the 2009 report on child protection by the Cour des Comptes, which called for the launch of research programs on the future of children in care, and the evaluation of policies and systems. These recommendations went unheeded.

In Conclusion

- given this Lilliputian budget - in the fields of medicine, child psychiatry, psychology, education or sociology, in order to improve their lot.

France, which led the way in taking in abandoned children between the 17th and 19th centuries, is now lagging far behind. Are we still the crucible of human rights?

Afterword

A brief history of the historical debate on children's right to attachment

The custom of "exposing" newborn babies, i.e. abandoning them in a public space - a form of customary infanticide - dates back to the earliest antiquity, particularly in Greek and Latin culture[64]. The other two sources of our Western culture, the biblical tradition and Egyptian antiquity, on the other hand, were repugnant to this practice. Although a number of charitable institutions appeared in Europe in the early 20th century to take in abandoned newborns, these experiments remained sporadic, local, urban and temporary until the 17th century.

---

64. BRULÉ (Pierre), "L'exposition des enfants en Grèce antique : une forme d'infanticide", *Enfances & PSY*, no 44, Érès, March 2009.

The situation gradually changed with the change in status of the "Maisons des Enfants trouvés"[65] at the instigation of Saint Vincent de Paul in 1638. The true genius of this man was to move abandoned children from private charity to that of the King, and therefore of the State. Using his influence with Anne of Austria, Queen and later Regent, he obtained a better fate for the children exposed to the law, who then changed their status and name: from then on, they were called "foundlings". As early as 1642[66], Louis XIII guaranteed subsidies for the "Maison de la Couche des enfants trouvés", dedicated to the care of these unfortunate children, for whom in 1670[67] (ten years after the death of Saint Vincent de Paul) Louis XIV reaffirmed

---

65. "As early as 1326, a hospice for foundlings (Les Enfants bleus) was founded in Paris, followed in 1537 by one for the Enfants rouges or Enfants Dieu. But it wasn't until Saint Vincent de Paul that assistance to children was truly organized", MARION (Marcel), "Enfants trouvés", in *Dictionnaire des institutions de la France aux xviie et xviiie siècles*, Paris, Picard, 1923.

66. Preamble to the letters patent issued by Louis XIII in 1642: "Having been informed by persons of great piety, that the little care that has been taken up to now for the feeding and support of foundlings, exposed in our good city and suburb of Paris, has not only been the cause that, for several years, it has been almost impossible to find a very small number who have been guaranteed death, but also that it has been known that some have been sold to be assumed and used for other bad effects [...]", TERME et MONTFALCON, *op. cit*, p. 99.

67. Letters patent from Louis XIV, June 1670, preamble: "As there is no duty more natural or more in keeping with Christian charity than to care for poor exposed children, whose weakness and misfortune make them equally worthy of compassion [...] Considering how advantageous their preservation is, since some can become soldiers, others workers or inhabitants of the colonies, we declare by article 6 of the regulations [...]".

and increased the State's financial commitment. The establishment became known as the "Hospice des Enfants trouvés", and was administratively attached to the Paris General Hospital[68], whose management was entrusted to the Jansenists, great enemies of Saint Vincent de Paul.

From then on, the children were visited by doctors, whose writings were added to over the following three centuries, providing invaluable evidence of the history of this institution, which preceded the organization of child protection in France. This edict of June 1670 prefigured the legal and institutionalized relief of foundlings after the French Revolution, which became enshrined in the laws of the Republic[69]. Foundlings became the responsibility of the State, which organized their guardianship, and of the hospital administration, which took care of them. The Emperor imposed these provisions throughout France with a new decree[70] in 1811, which established the widespread use of towers in every département - contrary to popular hagiography, it was not Saint Vincent de Paul who spread the use of "towers", but Napoleon I. This collection

---

68. "Ordonnons, dit le Roi, que la direction dudit hôpital des enfants trouvés sera faite par les directeurs de l'hôpital général, auquel nous l'avons uni et l'unissons par les présentes", royal edict of June 1670, *in* LALLEMAND (Léon), *Histoire des enfants trouvés et délaissés*, Paris, Picard et Guillaumin, 1885, p. 138.

69. "Law relating to abandoned children of 27 frimaire an V: Art. Ier. Newly-born abandoned children will be received free of charge in all the Republic's hospices."

70. Imperial decree of January 19, 1811:" Article 1. Children whose education is entrusted to public charity are: 1 - foundlings, 2 - abandoned children, 3 - poor orphans. Article 2. Foundlings are those who, born of unknown fathers and mothers, have been found exposed in any place, or brought to the hospices intended to receive them."

of foundlings, initiated by a charitable organization and then institutionalized by the State, profoundly changed the way they were cared for. Official statistics were then compiled to record the number of foundlings and the cost of caring for them.

On April 30, 1838, at the annual general meeting of the Société de la Moralité Chrétienne, Alphonse de Lamartine, then a member of Parliament, gave a speech *on found-lings*[71]. In it, he shone more for his qualities as a romantic poet than for his lucidity as a politician.

"Gentlemen,

When one of these poor children abandoned by misery, or whose birth is hidden by shame, is brought at night to the threshold of a hospice where he is expected at all hours, he is placed in a tower, an ingenious invention of Christian charity, which has hands to receive, but no eyes to see, no mouth to reveal. A tinkling bell announces that the tower has been visited. The pious sisters who watch over the walls rush to welcome the new guest. If he's naked, he's clothed; if he's covered in filthy rags, they're exchanged for clean, warm swaddling clothes. A nurse who has been housed and cared for by the hospice for several days is awakened and feeds him. At daylight, a healthy, robust woman from the fields, whose morality is attested by the magistrates, comes to fetch the infant, carries it on her shoulders and lays it in her own child's cradle. Beforehand, signs of recognition have been detached from the child, inscribed on registers, and will make it possible to follow its trail, if ever the circumstances

---

71. LAMARTINE (Alphonse de), *Œuvres I*, Paris, Gosselin, 1849.

that forced the mother to abandon it allow her to follow it with an unnoticed glance, and claim her son."

Lamartine could not have been unaware of the appalling mortality rate in these asylums. At the beginning of the 19th century, no more than one in ten foundlings made it past the age of ten, while more than seven in ten children raised by their mothers did. Over the period 1815-1848, i.e. thirty-three years, a study of the registers of the various hospices des Enfants trouvés in France puts the number of deaths among foundlings at one million twenty thousand nine hundred and seventy-seven[72]. This does not include babies who died in public spaces before being taken in. By extrapolation, we can consider that over the course of the 18th and 19th centuries, at least six million infants died in these asylums, a forgotten health catastrophe that mobilized hospital doctors.

French statistician and demographer Louis-François Benoiston de Châteauneuf, in his report to the Royal Academy of Sciences in 1824, concluded that "the abandonment of children by their mothers is in itself a more destructive cause of death than the two most cruel scourges that can decimate the human race, war and the plague".

Numerous writings and scientific works were then published in an attempt to "save and conserve this abandoned breed"[73], some of which were awarded prizes by several

---

72. *Monographie statistique et bibliographique des enfants abandonnés et assistés*, Paris, C. Renaud, Turpin et Juvet, 1864, p. 20.

73. NECKER (M.), *De l'administration des finances de la France*, 1784, tome III, p. 198, available on gallica.bnf.fr

academies[74]. In 1849, Ad. de Watteville had even compiled an abundant bibliography of over a hundred references[75]. Better rules of hygiene, the discovery of vaccination, natural breastfeeding and the decision to keep foundlings in the community for as short a time as possible, led to a gradual improvement in the "conservation" of foundlings. By the end of the eighteenth century, however, it had already been noted that advances in hygiene, nutrition and care were not enough to ensure the survival of abandoned babies, and that good emotional conditions were essential.

For example, Fodéré, a physician in Marseille, wrote[76]:

"Such was their lot, for the most part, at the Marseilles hospital, when I was its physician in 1796, and such had been their lot under my father-in-law, whom I succeeded. They were piled up in low, poorly-lit and poorly-ventilated rooms, which also served as stretchers for their swaddling clothes; the avenue of these rooms was occupied by small beers, sad omens of the end that awaited them; they were fed indiscriminately by mother-mothers, received at the hospital to give birth, on the condition, which was de

---

74. This non-exhaustive list of contemporary works on this drama includes: GAILLARD (Abbé), *Recherches administratives, statistiques et morales sur les enfants naturels et les enfants trouvés*, Paris, Leclerc, 1837. BENOISTON DE CHÂTEAUNEUF (Louis-François), *Considérations sur les enfans trouvés*, memoir read at the Académie royale des sciences, 1825, available on gallica.bnf.frArticles "Enfan trouvé et mortalité", in *Dictionnaire des sciences médicales*, Paris, Panckoucke, 1821.

75. WATTEVILLE (Ad. de), *Rapport à M. le ministre de l'Intérieur sur la situation administrative, morale et financière du Service des enfants trouvés et abandonnés en France*, BNF, Paris, 1849.

76. FODÉRÉ (F.-E.), *Essai historique et moral sur la pauvreté des nations, la population, la mendicité, les hôpitaux et les enfans trouvés*, Paris, Huzard, 1825, pp. 542-543.

rigueur, that they would not breastfeed their own child, but that their milk would be used to feed strangers, and that they would only leave this sort of prison after nine months. A single nurse served three, four, five, sometimes six children, among whom she could not recognize her own; a refinement devised to stifle all feelings of maternal love; so that each nurse was equal to all, and remained indifferent to the blows of the Fate, which often harvested around her ninety children out of a hundred of those received each year; and it was still the same in 1822, during a visit I made to this hospital."

This story clearly illustrates a twofold debate that remains unresolved over two centuries later, and constitutes a permanent stumbling block between professionals and managers, between the field and politics, between those who deal with the misery of children and those who finance their upkeep. Should society support or punish the parents of these abused babies? Should professionals remain aloof or allow these little beings to become attached to them?

However, the same observations were repeated over time. As early as 1815, Dr Marc[77] pointed out that "one of the main causes of the small number of foundlings that we manage to raise consists in the poor diet or deprivation of mother's milk", and that when they can be breastfed, we come up against "the indifference of nurses towards beings who are totally foreign to them".

And in 1840, Dr. Montfalcon, a doctor at Lyon's Hospices d'Enfants trouvés, wrote[78]: "Serving newborn babies is

---

77. Article "Enfan trouvé", in *Dictionnaire des sciences médicales*, Paris, Panckoucke, 1815, vol. XII, p. 279.

78. TERME and MONTFALCON, *op. cit.* p. 279.

Afterword

a much more difficult task than you might think; to do it well, it's not enough to have a sense of duty, you also need to understand and love children. Without a love of children, the nuns to whom they are entrusted in hospices will never perform their service well; zeal and exactitude, upheld by the Catholic faith, are invaluable qualities; but it's not enough if hospice sisters don't have that farsighted, vigilant affection for children, which no care or fatigue can deter. It has been rightly said that a mother and her newborn child, bound together by a holy tenderness, form the most harmonious being in nature; something of this maternal love is needed in the hospitable sisters who serve newborns. We've seen some excellent girls, but for whom this task was hardly appropriate; they didn't fail in any of their duties towards these little beings; they looked after them with intelligence, and yet something was missing: love of children: without it, exactness becomes routine, and routine leads to indifference. [...] Entrust two departments of foundlings, one to a hospitable woman who has only that banal charity for them which her habit makes her a law, and the other to a girl who naturally has a lively affection for them, and you will soon see the one keep a far greater number than the other."

Nearly a century later, in 1946, René Spitz, an American psychiatrist and psychoanalyst, put a name to the decline of emotionally estranged babies. He described "anaclitic depression" (partial affective deficiency) in children separated during the second half of life. When the separation was prolonged, there was an evolution towards a state of physical and psychic stagnation, which Spitz called "hospitalism" (total affective deficiency). Death then occurred in more than a third of children. The dissemination of this work led to improvements in the care of children in orphanages and institutions who, although their mortality may have remained higher than normal, no longer developed these historic and extreme symptoms.

After the Second World War, following in particular the work of Anna Freud[79] and Dorothy Burlingham[80] on the one hand, and John Bowlby[81] on the other, who had observed the fate of children raised in institutions, another challenge emerged, which is still relevant half a century later: to ensure that children raised outside their families do not develop personality or attachment disorders that are detrimental to them.

In France, it was Jenny Aubry - Élisabeth Roudinesco's mother - a psychiatrist and psychoanalyst, head physician at the Hôpital des Enfants malades, who, as early as 1946, pushed forward this reflection and a research program around the lack of maternal care at the Parent de Rosan foundation, an annex of the Saint Vincent de Paul hospice. Observing personality disorders in many of the babies placed there, she wrote[82]: "Many children arrive at the foundation for reasons that imply a previous life that was already abnormal: imprisonment or internment of one of the parents, parental decline, single mother, insalubrious housing or even homelessness, abandonment of one of the

---

79. FREUD (Anna), *Report for Unesco*, 1948.

80. FREUD (Anna) and BURLINGHAM (Dorothy), *Enfants sans famille*, Paris, PUF, 1949.

81. BOWLBY (John), *Maternal care and mental health, Report for WHO*, 1951.

82. AUBRY (Jenny), *La Carence des soins maternels*, Paris, Denoël, 1965, 2nd edition.

parents. It's easy to imagine the deficiencies and anomalies in the physical and psychological development of these children, shunted from hospital to institution, having received from their families only mediocre material care, little affection and in any case never any security or stability". She concluded her book with this painfully topical observation: "The fact remains that for children who have been deficient or rejected, the greatest danger is rejection."

In Hungary, pediatrician Emmi Pikler noted the negative effects of boarding school life for toddlers. She asserted that "even if the behavior of small children living in boarding schools of a relatively good standard can deceive a superficial observer, the majority of these children are seriously damaged from the point of view of their personality development". The rue Loczy institute, directed by this doctor from 1946 onwards, became a place of experimentation in personalized care for each child, which became a benchmark and was recognized by the WHO. Since then, many teams of professionals have been inspired by this approach in social nurseries and hospital wards.

Despite the sum total of these observations, and despite WHO's recognition of the need for this privileged, personalized care, the official discourse of certain political leaders[83]

---

83. Unfortunately, the conceptual advances made by childcare professionals in the field of childcare have not yet been taken up by politicians, who see this population as a source of endless expenditure - yes! resilience is also costly in hard cash - six billion euros a year for the French départements, according to the Cour des Comptes in 2009 - whereas Louis XIV saw it as an opportunity for the nation: "Considérant combien leur conservation est avantageuse, puisque les uns peuvent devenir soldats, les autres ouvriers ou habitants des colonies [...]", *Lettres patentes de Louis XIV*, June 1670, preamble.

or that of foster care or educational services remains crassly intellectually indignant, still denying children in care the right to become attached to the adults in charge of them, or reproaching these same guardian adults for having granted them this assistance[84].

All too often, the instructions given to foster families and educators remain to remain highly professional - that is, to remain impersonal and refuse to embody any emotional responsibility - in the form of an implicit injunction tirelessly repeated in various forms: "Above all, don't get attached to the children."

Stupid, murderous slogan.

---

84. On this subject, it's pleasant to read the outburst from the me-dia-savvy Bobigny children's judge, Jean-Pierre Rosenczveig, in his blog of February 5, 2011, http://jprosen.blog.lemonde.fr/ "One might even add that many people today must find it hard to look at them-selves in the mirror when they display as their daily reference values: respect for the individual, children's rights, human rights, etc.! And what are we to think, in this case, of the president of the General Council [...] who positions himself as a hard-line defender of the institution, like a banal company director endorsing his employees? He'd like to bring tears to our eyes by commiserating with him. It's like a dream. Was there at least a just reason for the little girl's departure from the foster family, beyond the more than dubious arrangements made? Yes, says the department! And they put forward as a strong argument that the B...rs were too attached to the child. No doubt they think, without saying so, that "reciprocally, the child is too attached to them!

APPENDIX

Maine-et-Loire children's home nursery operations

Here's a list of nursery professions, broken down by function. For simplicity's sake, the term *"educator"* is used as a generic term for the "mothering" function, which is in fact mostly carried out by highly experienced "nursery assistants". The term "famille d'accueil" (foster family) is inaccurate, as it refers to the profession of "assistant familial" (family assistant). But "famille d'accueil" has become part of everyday language, and is the term most often used.

The mothering function :
Nursery assistants, the linchpins of our work with children, are each responsible for one or two children in particular. Early childhood educators and specialized educators are also part of the team.

Foster families or family assistants, who are an integral part of the nursery's staff, welcome the child into their home and have the same role as mother(s). They bring the child to the nursery several times a week.

We can also mention the maids and night watchmen who are always on hand for the children, or the cooks and linen maids whose dedication is well known to all the children.

The educational function :
The educational function is represented by a small kindergarten and a small national education class. We are fortunate to be able to offer high-quality cultural and artistic activities at a very early stage, with a music educator, a gardener and pigeon fancier, and children's storytellers. Some parents are invited to take part in these activities.

The caregiving function :
is embodied by a team of nurses, nursery nurses, a psychologist, a pediatrician and a child psychiatrist. The presence of doctors in this nursery is a rare luxury in France.

The management function :
Is run by a department manager, with initial training as a nursery nurse, executive training and over fifteen years' solid experience. She is assisted by an assistant.

The children are not kept confined to the nursery, and as soon as their condition allows, they go to the day nursery, the day-care center or the school. If they're not too insecure about going out, they go on vacation, to the seaside, the mountains, the market, the zoo and the cinema, like all the children in the world.

ACKNOWLEDGEMENTS

Jean-Bernard G., Philippe D., Jean P., Ludovic de G., Claire H., Bruno C., Annabelle A., for their advice,

to Anita C., Jérôme G., Marie-Paule V., Lucie B., Christine L., Danièle C., Valérie L., Marie-Noëlle L., Gaëlle D., Serge and Astrid C., Sylvie G., Marie-Laure B., Nathalie B., Gwenaëlle R., for all the exchanges that nourished this book,

and to all my other colleagues at the children's home, I'd like to reiterate the pleasure and intellectual satisfaction I derive from working with them.

Table of Contents

Best sellers Max Milo Editions

Hitler's banker, Jean-François Bouchard

Confessions of a forger, Éric Piedoie Le Tiec

The Koran and the flesh, Ludovic-Mohamed Zahed

Governing by fake news, Jacques Baud

Governing by chaos, Collectif

A political history of food, Paul Ariès

Mad in U.S.A.: The ravages of the "American model",
Michel Desmurget

Mondial soccer club geopolitics, Kévin Veyssière

Putin: Game master?, Jacques Braud

Treatise on the three impostors: Moses, Jesus, Muhammad,
The Spirit of Spinoza

TV Lobotomy, Michel Desmurget

* 9 7 8 2 3 1 5 0 1 2 2 5 1 *